JASON VALE'S

5:2
JUICE
DIET

The Perfect Weight Loss
& Health Management Plan

First published in 2015 by Juice Master Publications.

ISBN: 978-0-9547664-6-7

www.juicemaster.com

Written by Jason Vale with acknowledged contributions.

Design, layout and photography by Lightmill Ltd.

Design and Layout of 'SUPER fast FOOD' pages PDS Ltd.

CONTENTS

THANK YOU...

THANK YOU to my lovely Katie for some of the beautiful wholefood recipes, taken from the main *SUPER fast FOOD* book. Thank you also for just being just the most beautiful person in the world.

THANK YOU to the dynamic duo – Alex Leith and Kirsty Heber-Smith – for the beautiful recipe photography, they look so good you could almost drink them! Special thanks to Alex again for what I think is an awesome book cover!

THANK YOU to Charlie Leith for the lovely illustrations, typesetting and for making the colour pages and recipes look wonderful.

THANK YOU to David Nelson for the beautiful way you have constructed the colour wholefood recipe pages and for finding that really cool font!

THANK YOU to Andrea Wells my lovely PA, who has gone over this book again and again and again. She has made sure that the shopping lists match the weekly juices and generally ensured nothing is missed!

THANK YOU to Carly, Andrea and Charlie for making sure this book has hit the shelves without any glearing spelling or grammatical errors (that was a joke, clearly I meant glaring!)

I'd like to also give a **THANK YOU** to the whole juicy team: from the people at Juicy HQ in the UK, the USA and Australian team, everyone who works at the retreats, the people who work on the Juice Academy, the Juice Master Delivered crew and all those who just believe in what we do and who care more for others than themselves.

THANK YOU, TEAM JUICE!

'YOU TAKE A PERSON,
YOU FAST THEM, AFTER
24 HOURS EVERYTHING
IS REVOLUTIONISED.
AND EVEN IF YOU TOOK
A COCKTAIL OF DRUGS,
VERY POTENT DRUGS,
YOU WILL NEVER EVEN
GET CLOSE TO WHAT
FASTING DOES.'

— PROFESSOR VALTER LONGO
(DIRECTOR OF THE UNIVERSITY OF SOUTHERN CALIFORNIA'S LONGEVITY INSTITUTE)

BEFORE WE BEGIN — PLEASE READ

A little note from the author...

It doesn't matter if you're a juice veteran or a juice virgin, anyone can reap the benefits of this *5:2 Juice Diet*. It is the perfect follow-on for anyone who has already completed one of my full-on Juice Diets. However, it is also effective as a stand-alone system for anyone who has no desire to ever go on a full-on juice diet. I understand that living on nothing but juice for five, seven, ten (or in some cases, 28 days), isn't for everyone. In fact it's fair to say that one of my friend's reactions to such a suggestion mirrors the opinion of many, 'I'd rather stick needles in my eyes'. His opinion is born out of never actually trying it and, should he ever take the full juice plunge, he's in for a very pleasant surprise. However, until someone has experienced it, it does sound, on the surface at least, something few would ever get excited about doing. However, when I mentioned this *5:2 Juice Diet* concept, he suddenly became interested. He has witnessed the incredible results juicing can provide, as he's not only seen the turnaround in my own health, but also in the thousands of people who have written to me over the years. Despite these changes, the thought of not using his teeth for a week to chew food and being on nothing but juice for that length of time, was about as appealing as a holiday in Iraq! However, when I mentioned I was writing this book, a plan where he would only ever go a full day without a meal, his ears pricked up. The thought of not using his teeth for just two days a week and, as those days didn't have to be consecutive, was something he was willing to try. To his surprise, not only did he love the juices (something he didn't think he would as they are full of vegetables, not his number one choice of food or beverage) but, as of this book being written, he's kept it up every week for the past twelve weeks and lost 16lbs. To his astonishment, he's found it easy and now even looks forward to his 'juice-only' days. He says he doesn't feel like he's 'on a diet' but rather it's become part of his diet. He says it's something he envisages doing for life (minus holidays, as he's pointed out!)

What is most surprising is that he's vowed to join in my next *Global Juice Challenge*, something I didn't think he'd ever do. If you're new to the world of *'Juicing With Jason'*, every year I run four *Global Juice Challenges*, usually for a duration of five or seven days. We have around 50,000 people from over 100 countries joining in and it's become the 'body service' of choice for many people, four times a year. I am a huge advocate of 'putting your body in for a service', as I'll explain later in the book. And doing a prolonged juice-only 'fast' for five days or more, once every season, is something I actively encourage everyone to do. The *Global Juice Challenges* came about simply because this is something I do myself and thought it would be cool to have people join in to help support each other. It simply grew from there – it is also a way to ensure I do it too! (By the way, in case you think I am selling you my *Global Juice Challenge*, it's always 100 per cent FREE to all and I'm there to guide you through *www. jasonvalesbigjuicechallenge.com*.)

Now at this stage, if you are new to any kind of 'juice fasting', you'll probably be in the same camp as my friend and, at this stage, you'll probably have more desire to French kiss a skunk than live on fresh juices for seven straight days. I am hoping that once you get used to the 5:2 juicy way of life, your thoughts will change and I'll be seeing you four-times-a-year for your seasonal 'body service'. In the meantime I need to convince you that juicing for two days a week is not only extremely beneficial, but also incredibly easy and a whole lot easier than you are possibly imagining right now. Unlike a full-on juice diet, there is no reason for the *5:2 Juice Diet* to interfere with your normal life and, in reality, like my friend, it can actually become your normal diet/life.

So whether you are brand new to all this or you're a diet or juice connoisseur, please open your mind and read the book. Please don't simply jump straight to the recipes thinking, 'I know all about juicing and the 5:2 principles, so I can just crack on'. The book is an extremely easy read and you may just pick up one new thought or concept. You've bought the book, so you may as well take the very short couple of hours it takes to read it and reap the full benefits of your investment.

Right then... let's begin!

'A LITTLE STARVATION CAN
REALLY DO MORE FOR THE
AVERAGE SICK MAN THAN
CAN THE BEST MEDICINES
AND THE BEST DOCTORS.'

— MARK TWAIN

REVOLUTIONIZING

THE
5:2
DIET

1

By now there's a good chance you will already be aware of the standard *5:2 Food Diet*, if not, here are the principles behind it in a nutshell. For two *non-consecutive* days a week, you are asked to consume no more than 500 calories a day (if you're a woman) or 600 calories a day (if you're a man). These calories can be made up of any food, a small burger, fries or even a coke, as long as it doesn't exceed the *5:2 Food Diet* daily calorie allowance for those two days. For the other five days you can eat *anything* you like.

The *5:2 Food Diet* isn't some crack-pot food fad that was dreamt up overnight, but rather a diet based around a fair degree of science on Calorie Restriction – which I will come to soon. However, like most things, I felt the *5:2 Food Diet* could be improved upon in two simple yet highly effective ways:

1. **What you consume on 'fasting' days**

2. **What you eat for the other five days**

I realise the appeal of the *5:2 Food Diet* way of life is not having to think about dieting or calories for five whole days a week and seemingly not having to think about healthy food...*at all.* However, as appealing as this is, it is flawed in the two areas I mentioned: what you consume for the other five days and, moreover, where your calories come from on your 'fasting' days. For the record, I will be putting the words 'fasting' and 'fast' in inverted commas throughout this book as a 'fast' is a period of time where *no* nutrition whatsoever is consumed. We are effectively 'fasting' every time we go to sleep and when we wake we break that 'fast', otherwise known as *break*fast. So, although I realise that technically you can never actually ever be on a juice 'fast', for the purposes of this book however, I will be referring to the two days on juice-only as 'fast' days (any pedantic people reading this will just have to get over it!)

If your aim is to be thin, irrespective of how healthy you are on the inside, then the original *5:2 Food Diet* could work for you (although, having said that, I know many people who do, despite what the inventors of the *5:2 Diet* claim, 'make up for lost eating time' during the five days they are allowed to eat whatever they like!) Thereby defeating the purpose! However, if your sole objective is just to get into those skinny jeans regardless of health, you may as well go on the triple C diet of cigarettes, coffee and cocaine – and achieve the same goal. Clearly I am being facetious (please don't try this at home, kids), but I have been writing about health/nutrition/juicing etc. for well over fifteen years now. The sole aim isn't to simply slip into those often illusive jeans, but rather to find a system that works, one where you can stay in those jeans whilst getting a good, solid amount of super nutrition into your system every week to keep you radiant and keep your immune system strong as an ox. This is where my new *5:2 Juice Diet* comes into play.

SIMPLE CONCEPT — INCREDIBLE RESULTS

The practicalities of the *5:2 Juice Diet* are ridiculously simple, but the effects it can have on your mental and physical health are extraordinary, especially given its simplicity. This isn't just hearsay either, the science on Intermittent Fasting, or Calorie Restriction is now pretty conclusive and more research is being done all the time as its popularity spreads. Calorie Restriction, in one guise or another, has been shown to improve mood, control weight, improve heart function, help to control diabetes, and improve memory. It also has a profound impact on longevity. I am yet to find a more effective way of maintaining weight loss than by following a complete juice diet and then following up with this *5:2 Juice Diet*. This is one of the areas where people struggle the most and I personally feel this could be a solution for many who may have 'slipped up' in the past. I will explain all of the potential health benefits in the *'why to'* section of the book, before getting down to the practicalities of the *'how to'*. On that note, just so you know where we are going, I have spilt the book into three main sections, with mini headings within those main areas. The three main headings are:

1. WHY

2. HOW (THE PLAN)

3. THE Q & A SESSION

I have concentrated the start of the book on the many reasons *why* you should make the *5:2 Juice Diet* a way of life, for the rest of your life. The reason for this is simple: the reasons *why* you should to do something will always far outweigh figuring out *how* you will do it. Without a strong enough *why,* chances are the *how* will become completely irrelevant, as you won't ever get to the point of following the *how* anyway. For example, when I bought an old derelict hotel in the middle of nowhere in central Portugal, I had no idea *how* I was ever going to turn it into a beautiful healing retreat where people would one day fly in from all over the world – but I knew *why* I had to do it. At the time of viewing the extremely run down property, my beautiful mother was coping with extremely aggressive stage-four lung cancer. At the time, although I really wanted to turn this place into somewhere people could come and heal, I couldn't figure out *how* I would ever be able to do it. I had no experience in turning an old hotel into a luxury health retreat, I didn't have the money to do so and all I could see was one almighty, seemingly impossible, task ahead of me. However, on my second viewing I took my mother with me and, just as I was veering heavily to a very clear, 'I think I'll leave it thank you very much', my mother created an almighty *why*. Her exact words were, 'Jason, this place is beautiful and it has an amazing healing energy about it. It's too late for me, but you have to build this so others have the opportunity to heal in this wonderful environment. This is the last thing I ask of you Jason, build it'.

This is what I mean by a strong *why*. I had no idea *how* I was ever going to do it; *how* I would ever find the money, *how* I would find the time, *how* I would find the right people, but the *why to* was so strong that my brain had to find a way, and it did. Juicy Oasis in Portugal is now one of the most highly respected health retreats in the world and my mother, I am sure, would have been extremely proud that it was transformed into exactly what she had envisaged. It was the same when I first started juicing. *Why* I needed to juice was what got me into juicing and what has kept me juicing daily since, not *how* to juice. Let's be honest here, *how* to juice is frighteningly easy. All you do is get some fruit and veg and pop it into the feeder of the juicer and boom – out comes freshly extracted juice. I don't mean to underplay it, but that's essentially it. Yes, you need to know what fruit and veg works with what, what you can juice and what you should blend etc., but once you've got the basics covered, unlike cooking, it's quite easy to master the art. It was reading about the incredible health benefits of juicing years ago that created a strong *why* I needed to juice, the *how to* actually do it inevitably followed.

My personal *why*, when it came to changing my diet and using juicing as the tool for doing so, was born out of my own ill health. I was covered from head to toe in psoriasis, I also had severe asthma, bad eczema, was overweight, had severe hay fever, smoked two to three packets of cigarettes a day and drank heavily. I also had no desire to eat anything that was remotely healthy. I knew instinctively that fruits and vegetables were the answer, but I hated them – I mean *really* hated them. I then read all about the power of juicing and the rest is history. The point is that it was the full understanding of *why* juicing was so good and *why* consuming fruits and vegetables in their raw state in the form of 'live' juice could potentially help all of my conditions, which lead me to want to find out *how* to do it. I haven't looked back since. Because I had a strong enough *why* I should get freshly extracted juice inside me along with the massive *why* I personally needed to do it, the usual obstacles of *how* to do it also fell by the wayside. Back then, even making a juice was a performance in itself and cleaning the machine was a nightmare. There were many reasons I could think of *why* not to do it, and making a juice and cleaning the machine was one of them. However, the second the reason *why* you should do it becomes more important than the *why* you shouldn't, it is then that the previous obstacles collapse in front of you – like cleaning the juicer!

Even today, when it comes to juicing, that is still people's number one bugbear. What I don't understand is that we have to clean everything, but because a juicer is a new item for many people, the cleaning of it gets a disproportionate bad rap. If you've ever done Jamie Oliver's *30 Minute Meals* (if you have two hours spare! – kidding Jamie... *ish*!) You will often be left with a ton of washing up. I think because making a juice isn't seen in the same way as making a meal, people feel the trade off isn't fair. However, compared to the daily nightmare of living with a chronic skin condition, along with severe asthma, eczema, hay fever and more back (and front) fat than you should ever see on a human, cleaning a juicer is nothing. Once I knew juicing would work for me, I jumped straight in and didn't care how long it would take to clean the machine. Luckily, 21st century juicers are now extremely easy to clean and please make a point of reading 'So What Juicer Is Best, Jase?' (PAGE 239/CHAPTER 10) at the end. Once I read the science and common sense logic of *why* plant-based food could and should also be used as a form of medicine, I was in. This was especially the case because 'genuine' medicine had completely failed me to that point. My *why* I should try it was as big as it gets. I certainly didn't have anything to lose by trying it, worst case, I'd get more fruit and vegetables in me than I'd had for many years. Luckily, for me, it worked on every front. My skin is clear, asthma gone, excess weight lost, I stopped smoking and I feel better today at 46 than I did at 26. I am not saying juicing is a cure-all, *but for me personally* it worked a treat on every level.

JUICE FOR LIFE
In Every Sense Of The Word

My desire for you is not to do juicing for two days a week for a couple of weeks and then store your juicer in the cupboard for it never to see daylight again. No, my aim is for you have a full understanding of *why* IF (Intermittent Fasting) or CR (Calorie Restriction) have such a profound impact on all aspects of mental and physical health. Once you do, the chances of you actually doing it, of it becoming part of your life for now and ever more, will increase exponentially. The science alone on CR and IF will create an incredibly strong *why,* as it's so compelling and hard to ignore, but once you add to that the huge health and weight loss benefits that freshly extracted fruit and vegetable juice can bring, you'll want to know the *how to* quicker than you can say, 'show me the juicer!'

And that is the point of this book, to get you to actually

follow through and try this baby on for size. Once you do, you'll be hooked. If you have read any of my previous books, you will know that has always been my focus. The truth is that the vast majority of cookbooks are used as decorative features on kitchen shelves, rather than as they were actually intended. The same is true of many 'diet' books. As a nation we are extremely good at buying them, but actually reading them and/or following through is another story. This is why I always focus the first half of my books on the *why to* and the second on the *how to*. I believe this is the main reason people get the results they do – because they actually read the book and get fully engaged and inspired, because of the *why*.

REAL RESULTS FROM REAL PEOPLE
The Best 'Why' There Is

Over the many years I have been doing this, I have seen some truly, truly remarkable health changes and 'dramatic weight loss results people' who have embarked on one of my full Juice Diets. I realise this will raise some sceptical eyebrows, particularly as you hear this so often in books of this nature. However, all I can say is I am not talking about just one or two emails here and there, or even a couple of hundred over the years, I am genuinely talking about thousands upon thousands of people reporting the same things. Even a few hundred I appreciate could be deemed as anecdotal, but thousands? At some stage surely it must shift from purely anecdotal to, 'let's pay attention here', especially when we are talking thousands of people from all walks of life, all over the world, reporting the same things. I often share these stories at various times throughout my books as I feel nothing inspires more, or creates a bigger *'why'* if you will, than hearing of the often dramatic changes of real people in the real world.

For example, in my last book, *Super Juice Me! 28-Day Juice Plan,* the *'why to'* jump-on-the-juicy-train practically wrote itself. This was because I decided to use the successes of others as the *why to* and inspiration at the start of the book. That particular book/plan came to life after a health documentary I filmed of the same name – *Super Juice Me! The Big Juice Experiment.* In the film I took eight people, with a number of different health conditions, and put them all on freshly extracted juices and green blends for 28 days. The results far exceeded even my own incredibly high expectations and the film has now been seen by millions of people from all over the world and continues to inspire people to better health. Because so many people had already been motivated by the movie and had, effectively, gone on to 'Super Juice' themselves by following the *Super Juice Me! 28-Day Juice Plan,* which I had already put together in an iTunes app. All I had to do was use their stories as the *why to* at the start of that book. I had literally hundreds of dramatic, life-changing stories to choose from. I knew that anyone overweight and/ or with health issue couldn't possibly read those stories without being inspired to give it a go. I vividly remember adding these incredible health transformations at the start of the book and thinking, 'why do I need to write the rest of the book?' – they were that powerful. On that note I would challenge anyone to either watch *Super Juice Me!* the film or read the opening to *Super Juice Me!* the book and not be inspired to incorporate freshly extracted juice into their life. I would go as far as to say, you wouldn't be able to watch the movie or read the book and not be able to manage at least one full week on pure juice. If you give someone a strong enough *why* to do it, the previous obstacles of *why* not to, no longer become an issue and you find the *how*.

CONSISTENT COMMITMENT
The Only Route To Lifelong Success

The first complete 'Juice Diet' I ever wrote was way back in 2006 and was entitled, *7lbs in 7 Days Juice Master Diet*. It went on to sell over three million copies, hit number one of all books on Amazon (the only juice book ever to do so), and it even knocked the *Da Vinci Code* off the top spot. Even to this day, it is constantly in the top five in its category. The reason I believe it has continued to be so successful is due to the fact it's not, despite the impression the title gives, a 'quick fix diet'. I made absolutely sure that the right psychology was included at the start of the book to enable people to not only complete the seven days, but more importantly, to use it as a launch to a complete turnaround in their health and weight. This is why I added a Phase Two and Three to illustrate the importance of how to reintroduce solid food after a juice-only diet and what to do in order to make sure the weight lost and health gained remained intact. To this day, I still get hundreds of emails each month from people all over the world who say that is precisely what happened after reading that particular book. Many report that the seven days of pure juice, along with *the right frame of mind and knowledge* the book provided, kick-started a health and weight loss avalanche, if you will, and enabled them to drop *all* of the excess weight which had plagued them for much of their life (not just the 7lbs in a week as promised in the book title) and regain good health.

However, as powerful as some of those changes were, maintaining that good health and body shape doesn't always pan out. For some, after the initial inspiration to do the seven days of juicing followed by a period of healthy eating and juicing afterwards, the junk food gremlin somehow starts to rear its ugly head again and Boom! You're back in the land of the fat and sick before you even know what's hit you! So whilst there are hundreds of thousands of people who have done one of my 'Juice Diets' and have gone on to maintain a healthy weight and good level of health by using the, 'what to do after your juice diet' principles I lay out in all of my books, there are of course many who find themselves back where they started before they even get the chance to say, 'Look I'm thin!'.

__IT__ ALWAYS WORKS — IF __YOU__ DO __IT__

So what makes the difference between the people who constantly succeed and those who fall by the wayside? Why does it ultimately work for some and not for others? The answer is simple, there is no *it* working at all. *You* are *it*. Either *you're* working or *you're* not. If *it* didn't work for you, it means *you* didn't work for *it*. I have not only written about this subject for well over a decade, but I have run 'juice-only' retreats for that long too. I have personally seen thousands of people from all over the world and I have yet to see *it* not work, even once. The *it* in question is a full 'juice-only' diet followed by consistent, daily juicing of some kind, along with consistent healthy eating and consistent daily exercise of some nature. The clue here is the word *consistent*. If you want to maintain good health and a body shape you're genuinely happy with, you need to incorporate what I call the CC approach – *Consistent Commitment*. It's the only way to have the same clothes fit you all year round and the only way of doing whatever you can to prevent getting sick. The people who say, 'Well *it* worked for me' are the people who apply the CC approach and the ones who say, 'Oh I tried that Jason Vale stuff and, like all other things I've tried, it worked for a short while. But then I just put all the weight back on again', are the ones who don't – it's that simple. All you have to do is look at the language used by so many people who blame everything else apart from themselves. 'Like all other things I've tried, it worked for a short while but then I just gained all the weight back again' You'll hear that a lot from people who refuse to take into account the possibility that maybe, just maybe, *they* might be the deciding factor here. They put the failure down to the diet, the system, the type of food, and so it goes on – they never think *they* have anything to do with it. The reality is there are two keys to ultimate success in this area:

1. Personal Responsibility

2. Consistent Commitment

It's the second one I am concentrating on for this book. *Consistently committing* to certain health habits on a daily/weekly basis. This is the ideal maintenance plan for a healthy weight and a healthy inside. *Constantly committing* to doing whatever it takes to create and keep those healthy habits for life. The aim of this book is to move you away from a 'binge health/binge disease' way of life, which is what so many people do. I know this as

I have been guilty of the same thing many times myself. The key is finding a way of life that works for life. That way of life also needs to take into account the 'being human' side of life, the side we all have that likes going out with friends and letting our hair, along with our eating rules, down a little. In other words, a way of life that doesn't always involve quinoa and a spiralizer for every meal! CC to a few basic health habits is all you need to do; you just need to create those habits. Once they are ingrained, they will become as automatic as brushing your teeth. Oh that has just reminded me of a recent television advert for Sensodyne toothpaste. A dentist comes on and talks about how people are saying that their sensitivity has returned despite using the toothpaste. He asks them if it worked at all, to which they reply, 'Yes when I was using it'. Their sensitivity only returned when they stopped using the sensitive preventing toothpaste. His advice? Carry on using the toothpaste! The toothpaste clearly works, but if a person stops using the toothpaste and their problem comes back, who is to blame? The toothpaste or the person? The answer is clear and I don't wish to treat you like a numpty, but you can see what I am getting at here. This is no more ludicrous than someone who uses a health and weight loss approach, which starts to work for them, who then stops it and says, 'It stopped working for me'. It is painfully clear, like the toothpaste, that *it* can and will only work if the person continues to *consistently commit* to using it.

Fresh juicing, healthy eating and exercise is the best fat loss and health 'pill' that you can take. Like with the toothpaste, stop taking the pill and the fat and ill health will always return. Imagine someone who is exercising daily and gets uber fit, then they suddenly stop exercising and become unfit. Now imagine how utterly insane it would sound if that person then started to say the reason they are now unfit is because, 'the exercise just stopped working for me'? Yet we seem to readily take someone's word that a certain diet or healthy way of eating just 'stopped working' the second they stopped doing it! MADNESS OF THE HIGHEST ORDER.

WHAT YOU DO <u>MOST</u> OF THE TIME

DETERMINES YOUR WEIGHT AND HEALTH

CC works both ways, positively and negatively. If you *consistently commit* to never exercising, *consistently commit* to eating crap food and drinks, *consistently commit* to bingeing then you will consistently get the results those types of commitments bring – excess fat, lethargy, ill health, self-hatred and lack of confidence to name but a few. However, if you *consistently commit* to exercising every single day, *consistently commit* to eating well *most* of the time, *consistently commit* to this *5:2 Juice Diet System every single week* and *consistently commit* to putting yourself in for a full weeks' 'health service' once every season, then you will consistently get the results those types of commitments always bring – a slim body, loads of energy, increased confidence, good health and the freedom to wear anything in your wardrobe, to name but a few.

On a personal level, because I have been there and worn the rather large t-shirt, and because the thought of heading back to the land of the fat and sick gives me the horrors, I now live by the CC system. I *consistently commit* to putting my body in for a service every season by *consistently committing* to four week-long 'juice fasts' a year. I am *consistently committed* to exercising for at least five days a week and I am now also *consistently committed* to doing the *5:2 Juice Diet every single week*, forever more. I *consistently commit* because, if I don't, I will get fat and sick again. I will most definitely be the size of a house in no time at all and covered in a skin disease and not able to breathe without drugs again. They say once you've been fat then it's easier to stack it on again, and I can safely say that's the truth. Some people have 'muscle memory', but I most certainly have 'fat memory!' Each decade your metabolism slows down by about ten per cent, so, at 46, my engine isn't running as fast as it used to and I need to take such changes into account too. This is why I am *consistently committed* to staying well as, if I don't, the only alternative is to *consistently commit* to being fat and sick.

You cannot simply sit on the fence with your weight and health; it really does tend to be one or the other. In the words from the movie *The Shawshank Redemption* it's a case of either, 'Get Busy Living or Get Busy Dying' – there's no in-between.

Yes there are some people who seemingly stay slim and healthy despite what they eat or whether they exercise, but these people are very rare, rarer than you think, and you just need to face facts: you're not one of them. If you were you wouldn't be reading this page of this book right now. No, it's not fair, but then staying fat and sick constantly saying 'It's not fair' won't change your situation one iota. I am hoping by the time you finish reading this book you will be making a solid decision to *consistently commit* to some new health habits rather than 'binge health' only to then 'binge disease'. I am hoping this is the catalyst for you finally getting off the crazy 'Diet Merry-go-round' and embracing something that works *consistently*. This is what most people's Yo-Yo Dieting life looks like… you may or may not recognise yourself here:

THE YO-YO DIET:

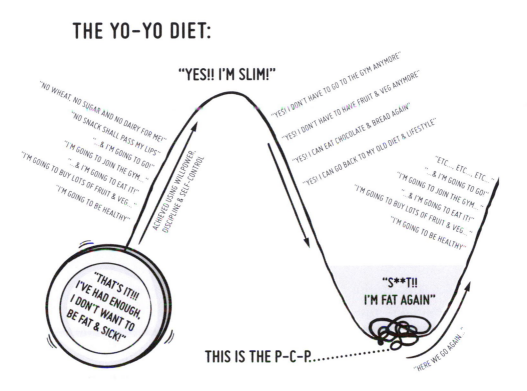

"YES!! I'M SLIM!"

"NO WHEAT, NO SUGAR AND NO DAIRY FOR ME!"
"NO SNACK SHALL PASS MY LIPS"
"...& I'M GOING TO GO!"
"I'M GOING TO JOIN THE GYM..."
"...& I'M GOING TO EAT IT!"
"I'M GOING TO BUY LOTS OF FRUIT & VEG..."
"I'M GOING TO BE HEALTHY"

ACHIEVED USING WILLPOWER, DISCIPLINE & SELF-CONTROL

"YES! I DON'T HAVE TO GO TO THE GYM ANYMORE"
"YES! I DON'T HAVE TO HAVE FRUIT & VEG ANYMORE"
"YES! I DON'T HAVE TO HAVE FRUIT & VEG ANYMORE"
"YES! I CAN EAT CHOCOLATE & BREAD AGAIN"
"YES! I CAN GO BACK TO MY OLD DIET & LIFESTYLE"

"ETC.... ETC.... ETC...."
"...& I'M GOING TO GO!"
"I'M GOING TO JOIN THE GYM..."
"...& I'M GOING TO EAT IT!"
"I'M GOING TO BUY LOTS OF FRUIT & VEG..."
"I'M GOING TO BE HEALTHY"

"THAT'S IT!!! I'VE HAD ENOUGH. I DON'T WANT TO BE FAT & SICK!"

"S**T!! I'M FAT AGAIN"

THIS IS THE P-C-P......

"HERE WE GO AGAIN..."

If this is not the first diet book you have ever read, then I am guessing you may well have recognised yourself in the diagram. When we hit what I describe as the P-C-P (Pressure Cooker Point) then, and only then, do we make a change. The P-C-P is different for everyone. For some it's when they have 10lbs of excess body fat and for others, their P-C-P doesn't kick in until they're 50lbs overweight. The P-C-P isn't just about excess weight either; it's when we reach a certain level of decline in energy/health and well-being in general. It's different for everyone and we all have our tipping moment into the *Pressure Cooker*

Point. On the bottom left of the diagram you'll see the sort of language used when one reaches their personal P-C-P:

'THAT'S IT! I'VE HAD ENOUGH.

I DON'T WANT TO BE FAT

AND SICK ANYMORE!'

This is the point when we say, 'Right enough is enough' and go into 'diet mode'. This usually involves using willpower, discipline and control for weeks on end, desperately denying ourselves the things we really want. It is this internal mental battle that sums up what I call a 'diet mentality' and is the main reason why people experience Yo-Yo Dieting. The P-C-P is when you start saying to yourself things like, 'Right, I'm going to buy some fruit and veg… and I'm actually going to eat it!' 'I'm going to join a gym… and I'm going to go!' 'No more chocolate, bread, pasta, sugar for me!' You get the idea. The P-C-P is not a half-hearted attempt to change; it's when you are *really* committed and ready to use whatever willpower and discipline you can muster to reach your goal. This is not to be confused with the fairly regular, 'I'm going to change my life on Monday' declarations that are made on an almost weekly basis. You know the times where you declare to yourself and your friends on a Friday that you're changing your life on Monday. The times where you go shopping for all your fruit and veg on the Sunday only to throw it all away on the Thursday as it's making its own way out of the fridge! The times where you join a gym, but end up paying for the most expensive sauna in the world, one you visit every two months! No, I am not talking the half-hearted 'On Monday I change it all' type declarations where you are secret eating by Wednesday and throwing in the towel come Thursday only to declare once again on Friday that on Monday you really mean it this time. I am talking about when you hit your P-C-P. It is obvious when you have – it's not a nice feeling and you want to do *anything* to move away from it. Let's just say it's the F word you want to move away from: FAT. You hit your *personal* P-C-P of fatness and start the journey. The problem is you tend to focus on what you *don't* want rather than what you do want. Most people say, 'I don't want to be FAT' rather than 'I want to be slim and healthy'. They tend to move away from something rather than towards something. You then 'white knuckle ride it' until you have reached your weight goal, or kind of reach it. On the diagram you'll see I have put 'YES, I'M SLIM... *ish'* as most people, when using sheer willpower, discipline and control, tend to settle for a goal which is slightly lower than the one they really want. You have created clear daylight between your P-C-P and where you are now, which means that, once again, you can feel a sense of relief that it's all over. You feel you have done extremely well and it's now time to reward what you perceive to be the hard work you've put in. It's at this stage the Yo-Yo Dieter tends to say things like;

'YES I'VE ACHIEVED MY GOAL! I DON'T HAVE TO EAT SALAD EVER AGAIN! I DON'T HAVE TO GO TO THE GYM ANYMORE! I CAN EAT BREAD AND CHOCOLATE AGAIN!'

Losing and gaining weight is a gradual process so it can take a little while before the effects of going back to your old ways shows itself as excess fat. It appears you wake up one day and the sudden realisation of slipping back hits you like a thunderbolt and BOOM! You look in the mirror and say, 'S**T I'M FAT AGAIN!' You have once again reached your P-C-P and off you go again.

STOP THE BINGE HEALTH/BINGE DISEASE MERRY-GO-ROUND

I have chosen FAT as the bench mark here but again, for you, it might not be and could be a decline in energy, health or general well-being that creates your P-C-P. There is nothing wrong with the *Pressure Cooker Point*, in fact, without it, you wouldn't make any change ever, it's the very thing needed to create enough pain for change. It's those who have gone past their P-C-P without doing anything who ultimately suffer the most. You see this in those weighing over 300lbs and those who eventually eat themselves to death. For whatever reason, they went past their P-C-P and just carried on eating. We have never had a time in human existence where we have so many people weighing 500lbs and over and where we have to take down walls just to get people out of their homes and into hospital. The mere fact you are reading this book tells me you are either at, or approaching, your P-C-P. Or of course, you have already been at your P-C-P and are reading this book after one of my full 'juice fasts' as a way of maintaining what you've already achieved. Ultimately, whatever camp you fall into, you are looking for a system that can act as a catalyst to lifelong change on the weight and health front, not just another start of the huge diet roller coaster. The only way to get off this roller coaster for life is to have a plan for life. It's all about adopting the CC (Consistent Commitment) methodology and doing something each and every week towards making sure you don't spring back. It's about creating lifelong 'health habits' that stick and following a system that works, not only on the 'staying in shape' front, but also on the 'being human' front. This is where I have failed personally in the past and is where a great deal of people mess up. Having smoked two to three packets of cigarettes a day, drunk my weight in alcohol every week and eaten junk food at every meal, why I ever thought my body couldn't put up with a *little* junk here and there when I went 'clean' I don't know. Flexibility is key to lifelong success. 'Being human' is key to lifelong success, along with the full understanding that in all probability you'll still, at times, have *slight* dips. What we are trying to do is move away from the *huge* dips that come with the usual Yo-Yo Diet (as illustrated in the diagram) and onto a life of *slight* dips which are easily countered.

CREATING A NEW P-C-P:

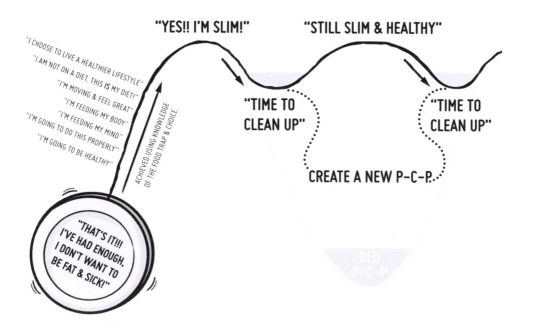

The aim is to create a new, much higher, *Pressure Cooker Point*. A P-C-P that automatically triggers a 'time to clean up' mode. My personal P-C-P is now set so high that it would be almost impossible for me to get that fat and sick ever again. If I do start to gain a little weight, for whatever reason, my new P-C-P level kicks in and my desire to *want* to clean up is almost instant. This is the key to lifelong success in this area, understanding that we all have a need to 'be 'human' at times, but to create an automatic 'clean up' trigger in the shape of a new P-C-P level. Funnily enough, as I write this section it is 'Results Day' at the end of one of my *Global Juice Challenges*. Someone has just written a post on Facebook that illustrates what I am trying to say beautifully:

'I use the scales at my local supermarket for a printout, these were broken. I drove to the next place I hadn't got the right cash! Then drove to town but it was so worth it! 1 Stone! 1 Stone! 14lbs in a week! I've been juicing for just over a year. Between May and December I lost 5 stone (70lbs) but I have been stuck and 5lbs crept back on! This week has kick started me. I'm now 3lbs off 6 stone. Soup 'n' Juice Me this week! Thank you so much Jason.'

— Lisa-Marie

The part I want you to concentrate on here is not the dramatic weight loss achieved in just seven days (although WOW!) and not even the incredible 70lbs weight loss overall, but rather, '... I have been stuck and 5lb crept back on...' Lisa-Marie has created an extremely high new level of personal P-C-P. Despite losing a massive 70lbs, the second just 5lbs crept back on BOOM! Her new level P-C-P kicked in and she went straight into 'time to clean up' mode. What the above shows is not just what juicing can do for long term weight loss, but once you create a new P-C-P and *consistently commit* to cleaning house the second it kicks in, you'll never return to the place from where you originally started. What this one Facebook post also illustrates is how powerful a full seven-day 'juice fast' can be. This morning I have read hundreds of posts like it and, once again, it only confirms everything I am writing in this book. Later I will be suggesting a way you can 'condense success' and launch yourself into the *5:2 Juice Diet* with such a bang that you'll be sold from the start.

The other key to lifelong success is to move away from a 'Diet Mentality' to a 'Freedom Mentality'. This is something I cover in all my books, as I believe it's fundamental, and I'll touch on it again here. It's a simple shift in mind-set, but one that's incredibly effective. It moves you away from the 'willpower and discipline method' to one of freedom where *you* are truly in control. It's where you stop saying to yourself, 'I *want* but I *can't* have', which is where people get stuck when using a 'diet mentality', and shift it to, 'I *can* but I *don't want* to have'. When I am doing my two days of juicing every week I am aware that I *can* have any food or drink I want. You may think I have lost the plot early on here, as clearly, I can't have anything other than the juices. However, what I mean is that I am an adult and I can have whatever the hell I like. I can have anything if I choose, but I am *choosing* to have the juices and *choosing* not have anything else. When I am on my two 'juice fast' days I have two choices. I can either put myself into what amounts to a 'self-imposed mental tantrum' and spend all day moping around for foods and drinks I hope I'll have the willpower to avoid, or, I can embrace the 'juice fast' days and understand at any given point I *can* have whatever I want. This is what causes more people to fail on any diet than anything else, the ridiculous situation where we spend most of the time dreaming of foods and drinks we hope we won't have. I can honestly say that by shifting from an 'I want but *can't* have' mentality to 'I can but I actually *don't want* to have' mentality, your two 'juice fast' days will transform from a white knuckle ride into to a breeze.

DON'T PLAY THE PERFECTION GAME

Above all though, what I would say is that in order to have lifelong success, don't try and play the perfection game!

YOU DON'T WANT TO SPEND YOUR ONE AND ONLY LIFE TRYING TO EXTEND THAT LIFE, ONLY TO FIND YOU MISSED IT TRYING TO BE PERFECT.

The Yo-Yo Diet Merry-go-round doesn't allow for 'being human'. It's all about being 100 per cent perfect. This is why I think so many people, having battled against a desire to have anything deemed 'naughty' for a significant length of time, rebel against it and then go on a junk food binge immediately after. This is also why, although I love the new trend towards pure health cookbooks, some of them don't allow for any flexibility at all and, in some ways, can add to the problem. Many of these books are all about being 100 per cent perfect, and *never* veering away from chia seeds, wheatgrass and cous cous! Yes, sugar, gluten, refined fats and the like are not good for us, but then I also think not 'being human' at times is equally not good for us either. I used to have no flexibility at all and didn't allow myself to be 'human' even once for many years. Yes I was slim and healthy, but would anyone ever invite me to dinner? It took me years to realise that if my body coped with all those cigarettes, that much alcohol and all the crap I poured into it daily, then I am sure a couple of 'being human' days a week wouldn't rock the slim and health boat too much. And it doesn't, the body is designed to cope with a certain amount of pretty much anything, but it's the *certain amount* we need to get right here! I believe that the *5:2 Juice Diet System* I have devised in this book is the perfect balance of health and human.

THIS 5:2 JUICE SYSTEM WORKS!
...BUT CLEARLY ONLY IF YOU ACTUALLY DO IT!

And that's what this is, more of a system, a way of life that allows for dinner parties and being social. However, it's all about the correct balance and unlike the *5:2 Food Diet*, I believe what you do for the other five days *does* matter. Having said that, if you've just picked up this book with the intention of living on juice for two days a week and having no 'food rules' for the other five, it will go a long, long way to maintaining your weight and health. The *5:2 Juice Diet* is incredibly effective even if the other five days go somewhat wayward. However, if you incorporate my *2:3:2 Juice Diet System*, explained throughout the book, you'll raise the game on every level and still have plenty of opportunity to be 'human'. On that note, that's the first thing to which you need to commit – finishing the book. Please do not make the mistake of jumping straight to the plan and just cracking on, **PLEASE READ THE BOOK FIRST.** Yes I appreciate that, like in all of my books, I rather annoyingly use twenty words where three would have done quite nicely, but my repetition is here for a reason. It is a form of conscious hypnosis and is very carefully designed to get into your subconscious, so you automatically act on the information contained within. And isn't that the whole point of this book, just to get yourself to act, to commit to get slim and well and to live there for life? I will never win any literary awards and I have no desire to. I just want people to get well and to not have to live a life of self-loathing, low confidence and constantly not being able to wear what they want. When I say to people that I write books they then return by saying, 'Oh you're an author'. But I am about as far away from an author as you can get. I write books but I am no author and I am not trying to be. I also don't care if anyone reading this finds it a little too intellectually beneath them. All my books are written in the same way, a way that is extremely easy and quick to read and is understood by *everyone*. So, given the nature of my deliberately repetitive writing, your commitment to read every page will probably be harder than the commitment to the *5:2 Juice System* itself!

LESS THAN A DAY TO

READ THE WHOLE BOOK

The good news is I have condensed the information to only include what I feel you need to know to inspire you do adopt the *5:2 Juice Diet* lifestyle. In reality, it will actually take you no longer than a day to read the whole book; for many people it will take no longer than an hour or two. I have kept the book 'lean' deliberately as I wanted to make reading it as easy as doing the 'diet' itself. So please take the small amount of time it will take to read the book as it may well provide that extra *why* that makes all the difference. It can make the difference between ending the Yo-Yo Diet Merry-go-round, or being caught in that pattern for life. To that end, and before we get into the *how* you make the *5:2 Juice System* a way of life, let's drill into some of the science behind the...

WHY TO 5:2?

THE 'SCIENCE'

'IF YOU TAKE MONKEYS, MICE, AND NOW WE'VE GOT A LOT OF EVIDENCE FOR HUMANS, TOO, AND YOU RESTRICT THEM CALORICALLY, NOT ONLY DO THEY LIVE LONGER, BUT THE PREVALENCE OF DISEASES GOES DOWN BY SEVERAL FOLDS.'

— PROFESSOR VALTER LONGO
(DIRECTOR OF THE UNIVERSITY OF SOUTHERN CALIFORNIA'S LONGEVITY INSTITUTE)

'THE SCIENTIFIC EVIDENCE
THAT INTERMITTENT
FASTING CAN HAVE
NUMEROUS HEALTH
BENEFITS IS STRONG.'

— PROFESSOR MARK MATTSON
(NATIONAL INSTITUTE ON AGING)

2

The ratio of 5:2 wasn't so much born out of science, but rather practicality, with a science foundation. It was Dr Michael Mosley who came up with the 5:2 concept after doing research into Calorie Restriction and Intermittent Fasting for a BBC television programme – *Horizon*. A great deal of the research had been done on ADF (Alternative Day Fasting) but not specifically on the 5:2 ratio. Alternative Day Fasting is, as the name suggests, where you 'fast' every other day. Dr Krista Varady of the University of Illinois at Chicago is one of the few researchers to have done actual clinical ADF trials on humans. In Michael Moseley's book, *The Fast Diet*, which later became better known as the *5:2 Diet*, he says that on 'fasting' days men should have 600 calories and women 500. This figure wasn't plucked out of thin air, nor did Michael come up with these numbers himself, but those numbers are based on the research conducted by Dr Krista Varady on ADF. On 'fast' days she asks her volunteers to consume just 25 per cent of their usual calorific needs. Woman are said to require 2,000 calories a day and men 2,500, so 25 per cent = 500 calories for women and roughly 600 calories for men. They are then allowed to eat whatever they wish on non-fast days. Dr Michael Mosley felt that the 'one day off' and 'one day on' way of life wasn't something he could ever do, as it would be, 'socially inconvenient as well as emotionally demanding' – and so 5:2 was born. By 'fasting' for just two, non-consecutive, days every week, rather than every other day, you can easily arrange your life around it – so I can see why Michael decided to adapt ADF into 5:2.

'Eight parts of a full stomach sustain the man; the other two sustain the doctor.'

— Japanese Proverb

Although the 'science' has been worked out at the 25 per cent of your usual calorie requirements, it doesn't mean that if you consumed 700 calories a day it wouldn't be just as effective. These are the numbers that have had some study at least on them so these are the numbers, like Michael Moseley, I am also sticking with. However, although Dr Mosley choose the 5:2 ratio for himself to fit into his lifestyle, the two days a week 'fasting' concept goes back way before his *The Fast Diet* book. Calorie Restriction as a concept has been around in one guise or another for thousands of years and it's far from new. Hippocrates was into it, Plato 'fasted' for greater physical and mental efficiency, many religions have some type of 'fasting' ritual as part of their faith – Lent, Yom Kippur, Ramadan etc. Calorie Restriction is also a philosophy the Japanese live by, *daily*. I also don't think it's coincidence that the Japanese happen to have the least amount of disease, the least amount of obesity and the longest lifespans of any other single nation on earth. Calorie Restriction, of some kind, is something they learn early and practice daily, particularly on the Island of Okinawa. It's something drilled into them as children. They even have a phrase for it 'Hara Hachi Bu', which roughly translated means 'Eat until you are eight parts (out of ten) full'. It is also often translated as 'belly 80 per cent full'. The Japanese are not in the habit of stretching their stomachs to capacity and they don't eat until bloated. They have an understanding that it takes around twenty minutes after eating food before the signal hits the brain that you've been fed and you feel fully satisfied. In the west we tend to eat until stuffed. The Japanese also don't 'snack' in the same way we do, instead they leave long periods between meals, allowing the body to fully adapt to and use the fuel that has come in. This is something we used to do in the west, but it is now a practice long forgotten. I see people now getting on a two hour plane journey, after already eating in the airport before the flight, chomping at the bit as soon as they're on board for the 'food trolley' to come round. It's a two-hour flight! It's worth also knowing that children now go an average of just one waking hour without some kind of 'snack' or 'meal' going into their mouths – that's just one hour. In the UK and good 'ole U. S. of A. we are about as far away from Calorie Restriction as it can possibly get and there is no question, we are fatter and sicker because of it, it appears we are also dying early because of it too.

In the 1930's biochemist Clive McCay, a professor at Cornell University, reported that significant Calorie Restriction actively prolonged life in laboratory animals. Authors Bradley and Craig Wilcox and Makoto Suzuke believe that *Hara Hachi Bu* may act as a form of calorie restriction, so extending life expectancy in humans. They believe *Hara Hachi Bu* assists in keeping the average Okinawan's BMI low, and this is thought to be due to the delay in the stomach stretch receptors that help signal feeling full. They believe that:

THE RESULT OF NOT PRACTICING 'HARA HACHI BU' IS A CONSTANT STRETCHING OF THE STOMACH THAT, IN TURN, INCREASES THE AMOUNT OF FOOD NEEDED TO FEEL FULL.

Over the years, there have been many experiments carried out in the area of Calorie Restriction, or Intermittent Fasting, and its effect on longevity. The vast majority of these experiments have been done on mice and, time and time again, show that Calorie Restriction has an almost astonishing effect on longevity. In one of the first books I ever wrote, going back over twelve years now, I talked about experiments on mice conducted by

Dr Roy Lee Walford. Dr Walford showed that by 'fasting' mice for just two days a week, *whilst making sure their nutritional requirements were also met*, you were able to double their lifespan. Mice live for roughly just two years, but, by using Calorie Restriction, that number was almost doubled. 'Fasting' has been proven to reduce the amount of IGF-1, an insulin-like growth hormone that your body produces. According to Valter Longo at the University of Southern California, less IGF-1, has been shown to reduce the risk of many age-related diseases. To test his theory, Longo genetically-engineered mice so that their bodies did not respond to IGF-1. He found these mice lived twice as long as the average mouse, and were healthy, when their calories were restricted. So if you want to eat a lot, the message is clear, consume *little* for two days a week and that way you may get to live longer and thus get to eat more in the long run!

In another study in 1945, mice were 'fasted' for either one day in four, one day in three or one day in two. The researchers found that the 'fasted' mice lived longer, *every time*. They also found the more they 'fasted', the longer they lived, which brings me to the point where, like anything, you can indeed take things too far. When I read, 'the more they fasted the longer they lived' I knew they didn't actually mean by not eating at all you'll live forever, I think we all know the opposite would be true there. Well, I say we all know the opposite would be true, but this seems like the perfect opportunity to bring up a movement that takes Calorie Restriction to the nutcase level – Breatharianism.

LIVING ON NOTHING BUT FRESH AIR

No I haven't just made up a word, it's actually a translation of the Latin word for 'fasting' – Inedia. Breatharians believe that it's possible for a person to live without consuming any food whatsoever. They even claim that food, and in some cases water, are not necessary for survival at all and that humans can be sustained solely by 'prana energy' alone – sunlight. The most famous person to expound the virtues of Breatharianism is an Australian woman who goes by the name Jasmuheen (although born Ellen Greve). Funnily enough, I wrote about her in my first ever book on food addiction, *Slim For Life – Freedom From The Food Trap,* explaining how bonkers, and dangerous, I thought she and her 'movement' was. In the 1990's, after releasing her book on Breatharianism, she made the somewhat unbelievable claim, 'I can go for months and months without having anything at all other than a cup of tea. My body runs on a different kind of nourishment. ' Because people didn't believe her, and why would you, she volunteered to be monitored closely by the Australian television program *60 Minutes* for one week without eating. However, Jasmuheen said she found it difficult on the third day of the test because the hotel room she was in for the duration of the experiment was located near a busy road. This apparently caused stress and pollution, which prevented absorption of required nutrients from the air. 'I asked for fresh air. Seventy percent of my nutrients come from fresh air. I couldn't even breathe,' she said. However, despite moving her on the third day of the test to a mountainside retreat, her condition continued to deteriorate, as it would! At least four of her followers have died as a direct result of her teachings, which comes as a shock to no one with even the slightest bit of common sense.

Clearly there's a balance to be had between, what I feel is the complete and utter nutcase Breatharian movement of Calorie Restriction (*zero* calories), and the situation we have in the west of never truly allowing our bodies to 'fast', other than while we are sleeping. The 5:2 concept of Calorie Restriction for two days of the week address that balance nicely for many people, especially if we're not going to adhere to the Japanese *Hara Hachi Bu* philosophy when we do eat. Like Michael Moseley, the thought of CR every other day, simply doesn't fit into my lifestyle. But I do agree that doing it for just two days a week has the potential to fit into most people's lifestyles. However, unlike the normal *5:2 Food Diet*, I am a firm believer that the quality of nutrition you take on board for the two 'fasting' days and what you eat for the other five days, *really, really* does matter (I'll be covering why soon).

ACTIVATING THE SKINNY GENE

This is the holy grail for anyone who wants to lose weight; to activate what's often referred to as, 'The Skinny Gene'. SIRT1, to give it it's actual name, is involved in the repair and maintenance of cells to promote survival during times of dietary scarcity. Wonderfully, SIRT1 also inhibits fat storage and is thought to deliver anti-ageing benefits to boot. If you are thinking about joining the *5:2 Juice Revolution* you'll be pleased to know that this 'Skinny Gene' is activated by IF (Intermittent Fasting) and CR (Calorie Restriction). This is made even better when combined with the DAF 16 (or 'Sweet 16') gene, which has been shown to switch on during 'fasting' tests on animals, keeping them younger for longer. So it appears IF has the ability keep us young and thin (where do I sign?!)

'FASTING' INCREASES THE EFFECTIVENESS

OF INSULIN, A HORMONE THAT

AFFECTS OUR ABILITY TO PROCESS

SUGAR AND BREAK DOWN FAT

The other thing you want to do in order to drop the excess bulge, is to increase the effectiveness of insulin. When we eat foods high in sugar and starches, it causes our blood glucose levels to rise. Our body produces the hormone insulin as a reaction to eating to keep our glucose (which gives our cells energy) from going too high or too low. It does this by taking some glucose out of the blood and storing it as glycogen in the liver, to be used later. Insulin also encourages fat cells to take up fatty acids and store them, the same way it encourages liver cells to take up sugars and store them. This is why insulin is known as the 'fat producing hormone'. Studies have shown that IF boosts the effectiveness of insulin to store glucose and *break down fats*, also referred to as insulin sensitivity. This is why IF can be so highly effective for weight loss, not just simply because you're consuming less food, but because of its insulin effectiveness.

If you only picked up this book as a way to lose weight and/or maintain weight you've already lost, you'll be pleased to know some other potential positive 'side-effects' of what you are about to embark on, all of which add up in the end to a very compelling *why*.

CR IMPROVES LEARNING AND MEMORY

BY STIMULATING NEW BRAIN CELLS

IN THE REGION OF THE BRAIN

RESPONSIBLE FOR MEMORY

In a study on mice, neuroscientist Mark Mattson found that IF increases levels of a protein called brain-derived neurotrophic factor, or BDNF. This, in turn, stimulates new brain cells in the hippocampus, the region of the brain that is responsible for memory. Mattson fed one group of mice a diet of junk food, while a different group of mice ate a low fat diet and 'fasted' for part of the week. **The mice fed the junk food became fat and had more problems navigating the maze to find food. The 'fasting' mice had more BDNF in their brains.** I call this the 'Limitless Effect' and something many experience when they come to the end of the full-on seven day 'juice fast'. The best way I can anecdotally describe it is a feeling of being charged, as if someone has literally plugged you in for a week. There is film called, *Limitless* where the main character takes a pill and becomes *Limitless*. He can write a book in days and learn a language in hours. Clearly living on juice for a week will not do such wonders, but you do feel Limitless. Not only do you feel great on a physical level, but your mind turns razor sharp and you have such clarity. After reading a little on the science of CR, I can only make the assumption that two things have happened. One, the 'junk food fog' that many go through life unaware of, has been lifted and two, there is more BDNF present in the brain.

NO FOOD CAN IMPROVE YOUR MOOD

If the potential of getting thinner, mentally sharper (as well as 'younger') aren't enough for you to adopt the *5:2 Juice Diet* for life, then hopefully the promise of a better mood might tip the balance. The protein BDNF has also been shown to suppress anxiety and elevate mood. During his experiments on IF on rats, Mark Mattson showed this to be true. He injected BDNF into their brains and it had the same effect as a regular antidepressant. This experiment hasn't been performed on humans, but people who have done the *5:2 Juice Diet* have reported better sleep patterns, increased mental clarity and better mood. It's worth pointing out here that if you eat extremely badly before embarking on the *5:2 Juice Diet*, then you will most likely experience 'withdrawal' from caffeine, refined fats and sugars. This can result in 'moodiness', rather than an improvement in overall mood. When your brain and body get used to living on juice for two days a week, your overall mood should then improve.

These are powerful and compelling reasons for doing Calorie Restriction and, in particular, due to the way it fits into your lifestyle, adopting the 5:2 approach of CR. However, as I mentioned at the start of the book, there are flaws with doing the *5:2 Food Diet*, none more so than what you consume for the other five days and the quality of nutrition on 'fasting days'. You have read above several reasons *why* 5:2, but now the question is...

WHY TO 5:2?

THE NUTRITION FACTOR

3

I have been doing some kind of Calorie Restriction Juice programme for the past 15 years now, starting my juicing life with a 'juice fast' lasting three whole months – yes THREE MONTHS on nothing but juice. I had no idea what I was actually doing and I was essentially the 'Juice Novice', but I was desperate to get well and had just read a little book on juicing and instinctively knew this was the answer. I hated vegetables; I mean really hated them and would never, ever eat them. I knew my 'beige and white food' diet was the caused my ill health, despite what any of the doctors at the time were saying It seems strange that, despite being covered in an extremely painful and horrific looking skin disease, taking an asthma pump up to 14 times a day, taking drugs for severe hay fever, that my doctor didn't mention diet as a possible cause, not even once! To this day many doctors, including one of the main media doctors on the BBC no less, still maintain that a change of diet does nothing for skin conditions or asthma. I find this not only frustrating, but incredible to think that some medical minds of the 21st century can dismiss the idea that diet can play a major role in fixing ill health. It is even more frustrating when these minds readily acknowledge that the *cause* of many health conditions are indeed diet related, yet refuse to consider a change in diet to be a cure for the same health conditions. Even the WHO (World Health Organisation) readily states that 85 per cent of all disease is caused by what humans consume, whether that's food, drink, cigarettes or drugs, so it stands to common-sense reasoning that a great deal of disease can indeed be helped by changing from a 'grey' diet to one of 'colour and life'.

This is why I *intuitively* knew that a change of diet was perhaps the answer, which led me to read this little juicing book to start with. Once read, it was crystal clear that turning fruits and vegetables into juice was indeed going to be the solution for me. There were two reasons why I knew this approach would work:

1. **I hated** raw vegetables and so would never have eaten them

2. The nutrition in juice is more bio-available than the whole food

The first was the biggest reason for me. I was addicted to white/beige food and nothing with any life or real goodness would ever enter my body. I didn't realise at the time that over 85 per cent of all fruits and vegetables were pure liquid and it was this highly nutritious liquid element of plant food that was the actual food part. Fibre cannot penetrate through the intestinal wall and it is only the *juice* contained within the fibre that feeds you. This liquid nutrition is more bio-available to the cells, meaning more of the nutrients contained with the raw fruit and vegetable gets to where it's most needed. I sensed my body needed a *lot* of extremely good nutrition in the fastest possible time and most effective way, and so juicing made a lot of sense. I then went to a health seminar and heard that a prolonged 'juice fast' would be the answer to clear my psoriasis, so I *immediately* put it into action. I now had an extremely powerful *why* this was a good idea and I was desperate to clear my skin. The problem was I was limited in what information was out there at the time and so I blindly juiced what I thought, and read, were the most nutritious – carrots. I read in the little juicing book I had that 'carrots were king' and why they were so good for in juice form. I even read about a man who had lived on carrot juice for a year and cured his cancer – so I was sold. Looking back with the knowledge I have now, living on virtually nothing but carrot juice for three months wasn't exactly the best idea I've ever had. In fact I know this to be the case as, at the end of the three-month 'juice fast', I was painfully thin and completely orange! My skin disease was also still there. My asthma had massively improved though, so I hadn't lost all faith. It was also clearly effective for weight loss, too effective it seemed, when you're on it for that long. However, despite my skin condition remaining and looking somewhat gaunt and unhealthy, I still felt there was something in this and perhaps I needed more than just carrot juice. I went onto read over 300 books on health and nutrition and I attended countless health seminars. The conclusion was clear, plant-based food, consisting of *numerous colours*, appeared to be the answer to a great deal of health issues. The missing link was the *numerous colours* part, not just orange. In fact, knowing what I know now, I cannot believe I did a full three months with no green juice at all, no wonder it had little effect. I also didn't include any fats during those three months, so it was always going to be impossible to clear my skin without those. Once I included different colour juices, added in some avocado and started to master the art of juicing, *everything* improved.

THE BIG JUICE EXPERIMENT

I conducted several 'juice fast' experiments on myself to see what was most effective and changed ingredients and the times I would drink the juice accordingly. I got my friends to try my seven-day 'juice fast' I had devised and the results were off the scale. This was of course back in the day way before everyone and their mother was coming up with 'juice cleanses'; this was *real* and born out of my frustrations with my own health. My seven-day 'juice fast' also wasn't just thrown together, it was, and is, an extremely well thought through, tried and tested, juice plan. Once I had it just right and knew the results people would get, if I could just convince them to do it. I launched it as book – *7lbs in 7 Days Juice Master Diet* – and the rest is history.

Since those early 'juice fast' experiments, I have spent my life trying different ones and being my own constant guinea pig. 'Juice fasting' is something I feel I have majored in, been there – seen it – done it and very much worn the 'juice fast' t-shirt. For me it doesn't have to just sound good in theory, it has to work on a huge scale, where the results surprise and blow people away. This is why I have completed my own *Super Juice Me! 28-Day Juice Fast* – twice. I did it once when filming the documentary *Super Juice Me! The Big Juice Experiment* and another time in January 2015. I had no intention of doing it twice, but I was under pressure to 'prove' I could do it away from the comfort of my retreat. *Super Juice Me!* was filmed at my retreat in Portugal and I did the 28 days along with, what are now referred to as, the *Super Juicers*. All of our juices were made for us and we were in a 'locked in' environment in the middle of nowhere in Portugal. Because people tend to look for any excuse as to why they wouldn't be able to do it, the one which sprung up for many was that, 'Well anyone could do it on a retreat'. They often expressed this opinion with a little anger, as if I was wrong to suggest it was possible to do this at home, when working in a cold environment surrounded by friends etc. etc.. Many either didn't know, or had forgotten, that I once did three whole months at home, whilst working, surrounded by friends etc. on pure juice-only, but they wanted me to prove I could do it *away* from the retreat.

THE ULTIMATE 'JUICE FASTING' GUINEA PIG

What many didn't realise was that in a six-week period leading up to the filming of *Super Juice Me!* I decided to super size myself. I did this so that people couldn't say that it was different for me because I wasn't 'coming off junk food' or that I wouldn't have any 'detox symptoms'. I also wanted to *be* with the people taking part in the experiment, I mean really *be* with them on every level. So for six weeks I ate my way to being a little fat camper again. Like I said earlier in the book, my 'fat memory' is pretty amazing and I stacked on over 30lbs in those six weeks. People ask what did I eat during that time, the answer – everything! What was interesting was to see how rapidly not only the weight piled back on again, but how my breathing started to become extremely shallow and how unfit I got (I also made a point of not exercising during that time, which for me was a nightmare!) I was also shocked to see how quickly that 'addiction memory' kicks back in. I reached the stage where I was starting to get a drug like high from the 'foods' and 'drinks' I was having. Moreover, I started to get the fear of not having them, which is *the* sign of addiction! After three days the 'withdrawal' from the junk had gone and in the 28 days I dropped the whole excess 30lbs and actually felt better than I did before I started the whole experiment. People think I live on juice all the time and that's far from the case, so when I went for 28 days straight on juice, I felt truly amazing. I then decided to repeat the whole experiment at home, in January 2015 as mentioned, for the reasons given. When I say I decided to repeat the whole experiment, I mean *exactly* as I did it the first time. That meant putting my body and mind once again through the mill by super sizing myself. Once again, frighteningly easy to pile the weight back on due to my incredible 'fat memory' and, once again, the addiction gremlin came to say 'Hi!' In fact, this time, I managed to balloon to a whopping 189lbs (13.5 stone), I know! I knew I had a very, very busy January and so it would be an ideal time to prove to the naysayers that, if you are committed, it can be done no matter what time of year it is or what you have on. Not only was I running '*The World's Biggest Juice Detox*' for the whole month, but I had loads of TV, a new book launch, Ireland premiere of the film and my first seminar in London for over six years. Over 1000 people came to *Super Juiced! The Seminar* and I was on stage for over seven hours. I then had a two hour book signing afterwards and was extremely tired by the end. At this stage I was on day six of my *28-Day Super Juice Me!* in the real world experiment. Trust me, after a day like that; the last thing I wanted to have for dinner was a juice in my hotel room! However, I was completely committed and so stayed firmly on the plan. I then had to get up at 6am for morning TV, so if anyone says I don't know what it's like to do that kind of 'juice fast' in the 'real world', I think during the mad month that was January 2015, I proved that is far from the case. Once again I dropped over 30lbs and felt amazing.

5:2 JUICE DIET FOLLOW ON

This is when I decided to commit to two days of juicing every week for the whole of 2015. My fat memory, due to the 'juice fast' experiments I was putting myself through, seemed to be getting a memory that even the wonderful Stephen Fry would be proud of – so I wanted to make sure that I was equally committed to this. I also wanted to see what the effects of the *5:2 Food Diet* would be with juice. One thing is clear, by juicing for two days every week, eating and juicing well for at least three of the other five days and doing four full 'juice fasts' a year, seems to be the holy grail of weight loss and health management. I say the holy grail because it allows for the human side of 'being human'.

WE ARE NOT BONOBO CHIMPANZEES!

For many years I was incredibly strict with my diet, to the point where I had stopped 'being human'. Friends would stop inviting me out for dinner because I was such a pain in the arse, which I was! I wouldn't even have tea or coffee in the house and only offered people herbal teas. Every time I went to a restaurant I would ask where everything had been grown, I was starting to bore myself. I always mentioned to people that our closest living relatives are the Bonobo Chimpanzees and how they are 99.9 per cent genetically the same as humans and all they eat are green leaves and berries. What I hadn't appreciated was that although there was only 0.1 per cent difference in our genetics that 0.1 per cent, it turns out, makes quite a big difference. That 0.1 per cent means the bonobo isn't particularly good to play chess with and not the best guests at a dinner party! I went from being completely unbalanced for many years in the junk direction to being, what I feel, was completely unbalanced in the health direction. This is why I now live by and love *this 5:2 Juice Diet*. The one I have devised doesn't simply involve juicing for two days and going mental for the other five, which is where I feel the *5:2 Food Diet* is flawed, but gives a more balanced approach to both camps. It allows you to be 'human' and have dinner parties, whilst at the same time guarantees in the first instance, weight loss, (if you need to) but then to maintain the weight lost. This *5:2 Juice Diet* also *heavily* takes into account the nutrition side of life, guaranteeing you get a level of *genuine live* nutrition each and every week that most simply never get to achieve. It also guarantees the many benefits Calorie Restriction and Intermittent Fasting has to offer, but, I feel, in the correct way by taking into account the 'nutrition factor'. I can honestly say that if I didn't juice I would never get the regular quota of fruits and vegetables into my system. There is certainly no way I'd get the variety I do, or the spectrum of colours. You can consume the nutrition of many different fruits and vegetables in one hit when you juice and I, for one, would never sit down and eat a plateful of ten different *raw* vegetables. Yes my taste buds have changed a little and I have grown to love far more vegetables than I ever did, but the idea of a plate of raw broccoli and cauliflower still doesn't have me doing cartwheels! Whereas juicing the vegetables and mixing them with a little apple, pineapple, ginger, lime or mint and I'm in! My theory was, 'If you can't eat vegetables, drink them.' And that is what I have been doing for the past 15 years, drinking shed loads of different coloured fruits and vegetables *daily*. I now drink *nothing* but juice two days a week, but still have at least one vegetable packed juice for three of the other five days and I eat 'clean' for three of the other five days.

I don't want you to be *on* the *5:2 Juice Diet* but rather for it to *become* your diet. I feel this lifestyle is achievable for most and once you've done it for a while, it just becomes 'what you do' and you don't even think about it.

THE 5:2 JUICE SYSTEM

The book is entitled, The *5:2 Juice Diet*, but in reality it's more of a *2:3:2 Juice System*. If you apply the principles of this, *2:3:2 Juice System*, it will be *much* more effective than the usual *5:2 Food Diet*. It will go like this:

2 Days A Week = <u>PURE</u> JUICE

3 Days A Week = <u>PURE</u> FOOD & JUICE

2 Days A Week = ANYTHING THAT FLOATS YOUR BOAT!

This, as mentioned, is the ideal and I will explain fully what the system should look like on each day in a second, however, if you have picked up this book wanting do two days juicing and consume whatever you like for the other five days, then you are free, of course, to do that. The *5:2 Juice Diet* is clearly effective on just that basis alone as it guarantees an enormous amount of pure, raw, genuine 'live' nutrition going into your body for at least two days a week. It's worth pointing out at this stage that many people go days and sometimes weeks without having any fruits and vegetables in their raw and most nutritious form. Because the calorific value of the juices have also been worked out for you, there's no confusion or weighing and measuring, unlike the *5:2 Food Diet*. To be clear again on the calorie point, in case any pedantic science geek or doctor is reading and trying to catch me out (they do, I get the emails!), although some studies on ADF (Alternative Day Fasting) have been worked out using 500 calories a day for women and 600 calories a day for men, it doesn't mean that if both men and women consumed 700 calories each on 'fast' days that it wouldn't be equally as effective. If you know my work you will know that I hate the 'counting calorie' model with a passion and it's alien for me to be using it any way now. The *only* reason for doing so is that there has indeed been some research on these numbers and they do work, so in my head, why mess with it? It could be argued that I have messed with it slightly as on my *5:2 Juice Diet* both men and women have between 500/600 calories a day – the same amount for each gender – but this small shift will not make a jot of difference to the results. I know this as my *5:2 Juice Diet* app has already been out for eight months and I've had more than enough feedback to confirm this. So if you simply wished to adopt the principle of juicing for two days a week and sod the rest of the days, you'll still reap many benefits. Having said that, I am a firm believer that if you're going to do something, do it right. The whole point of writing this *5:2 Juice Diet* book is to revolutionise the *5:2 Diet* by improving the quality of the nutrition consumed on 'fast' days and to massively improve what you eat for the other days, hence the 2:3:2 adaptation (from this point on when I talk about the *5:2 Juice Diet*, you know I am referring to this 2:3:2 adaptation).

The reason I didn't make it two days *pure* juice and five days *pure* food is because that isn't a reality that many would ever fully adhere too, nor should they in my opinion. I have already mentioned we're not bonobo's and, if you're like me, you'll love dinner parties and letting your hair and 'food rules' down. On a personal level, I tend to 'loosen my food rules' at weekends and also on 'airport days'. Funnily enough, I am writing this page of the book whilst at an airport on my way to my retreat. A woman has just come up to me and said, 'Sorry to interrupt, but I had to come and say hello because you've changed my life and I want to say thank you.' She then went on to say, 'I don't drink coffee any more because of you' at which point I could feel her staring at the cappuccino I had in front of me! I didn't drink coffee for many years; in fact I didn't have anything other than 'clean' foods and drinks' for many years. These days I have found a balance that works on every level for me, including having 'airport days' which now and then includes the odd cappuccino. Two days of the week I'm on pure juice, three days I'll have juice and 'pure' food and at the weekends whatever takes my fancy! Well sometimes those three days turn into two and half days (well it's Friday night after all!) I have found that this balance fits perfectly into my world and I know from feedback and experience that it's a system that can work for most. I also, as I have expressed many times throughout this book, do at least four *one week* 'juice fasts' a year. You would never think of not servicing your car and it astounds me that some people never put their body in for a service. Your body is the most precious vehicle you'll ever own and, in today's over-polluted and hybrid food world, we need regular servicing more than ever. This is why I put on a totally free and guided 'juice fast' every season, starting with *'The World's Biggest Juice Detox'* every January and then three times a year we hold, *'Jason Vale's Big Juice Challenge'* (hope you'll start joining us) *www.jasonvalesbigjuicechallenge.com.*

The key here of course is not to simply adopt *this 5:2 Juice Diet* until you've dropped all the weight you need, to feel great and then celebrate by going back to the same old pattern of eating and drinking which led you to pick up this book in the first place. The whole, massively repeated theme throughout this book is to hammer home just how vital *Consistent Commitment* is for the lifelong success you're looking for. We need to move away from, 'Binge Disease – Binge Health – Binge Disease' and do something, *consistently,* that will keep us in the shape and health we want to have. You don't want to ever have to think about *if* a certain item of clothing you want to wear will still fit; *if* you can go to the beach; *if* you can sunbathe without feeling paranoid; *if* you are slowly poisoning your system; *if* you might get diabetes; *if... if... if... if...* you want to be free of all that and *know* you're good to go, always!

As I pointed out in the Yo-Yo Dieters diagram earlier, there will still be 'blips' – no matter how consistent we are there are always 'blips' – the key here is to make sure those tiny blips are just that, tiny blips. Yo-Yo Dieters don't have tiny blips, they have massive waves of the 'Binge Disease – Binge Health – Binge Disease' cycle. That's usually because they are trying to be too strict for too long and don't have 'human days' or 'human moments', this *5:2 Juice Diet* allows you to be 'human'. I remember my aunty Hilda making a beautiful homemade cake when I was in my, 'being perfect on the diet front' years. I said I'm sorry aunty but, 'I'm sugar-free, dairy-free, wheat-free, gluten-free, refined fat-free and additive-free' In reality I was personality free! I used to smoke two to three packets of cigarettes a day, drink over ten pints of beer daily, eat nothing but junk and yet I still lived. This proves that whatever we throw at the body, it has an ingenious filtration and a 'detox' system that does whatever it can to keep us alive. Clearly, at the rate I was putting crap, nicotine, smoke and alcohol into my body, I am unsure the filtration and natural 'detox' system would have continued working. In fact it clearly was showing signs of being under massive strain by the fact I was covered in a skin condition, couldn't breathe properly without the aid of medical drugs and had more excess fat than any chap should have on their body. Your natural filtration system will only last so long before it totally shuts down and can only handle a certain amount of toxicity coming into the body each day. However, when you eat 'clean' for *most of the time*, then it really can handle a slice of aunty Hilda's cake! Why I thought at one stage in my life that my body could easily deal with all those cigarettes, massive amounts of junk food and pints of alcohol daily, but would buckle under one single slice of cake is beyond me. I went from one end of the scale to the other and didn't give my body credit for the fact it was designed to deal with a certain amount of 'non ideal' foods and drinks for survival purposes. It's all about what you do *most* of the time and I believe my *5:2 Juice Diet* is something most people can do most of the time. I map out a 'rough' idea of what your non 'juice fast' days may look like soon. This will of course vary from person to person, but I think it's important to have a rough overview that you can incorporate into your own lifestyle and personal tastes. However, before I do and before you embark on the juicy 5:2 way of life for life, I'd like to do my best to try and persuade you to...

START WITH A BIG JUICY BANG!

If you are new to 'juice fasting' or not, one thing I would like to *heavily suggest* before adopting this *5:2 Juice Diet*, is to kick things off with a five day full-on 'juice fast'. Clearly you don't have to, nor need to do this, and you can just start with the *5:2 Juice Diet System* and all will be well, but I want to point out that if you do, it will actually make your journey into the *5:2 Juice Diet*, *easier*. That may sound crazy, but by kick starting your *5:2 Juice Diet* with a full five-day 'juice fast' you'll be totally convinced of the concept and you will start with a bang. You can read all about juice, the benefits, the rapid healthy weight loss, but nothing, I mean nothing, can actually prepare you for how you good you feel on the morning of day six after a full five days on juice (with no cheating!). Nothing can also prepare you for the amount of weight you can drop in that time either, and nothing is a more powerful convincer that fresh juicing works than doing a five-day 'juice fast'. The reason I am suggesting the five-day one and not the seven-day one, is so it still fits into the 5:2 model, only here it's five days on juice and two days on food. It means you still have your weekend and, if in the right frame of mind, should be far easier to do than you can imagine. You then kick off with the *5:2 Juice Diet* the following week. I have tried this with a few people and what it does more than anything else is give them such momentum that they want to and are itching to do the *5:2 Juice Diet*.

It is reported that the space shuttle requires 90 per cent of its energy just getting the space craft into space, it only requires ten per cent to keep it up there. See the five-day 'juice fast' as your launch into this. It may require slightly more energy to get you there, but once you arrive the following week, knowing you only have two days on juice, it all of a sudden feels easy. And that is what I want, for it to feel easy for you in the quickest time so that it really does become something you do consistently. Plus if you've had five days making juice and cleaning your juicer, two days will again seem a piece of cake. If you are new to juicing, this is also a good idea, as after five-days of consistently making juice, you become a master of the juice in no time. To wet your juicy appetite and to add weight to your *why*, you should perhaps think of doing a five-day 'juice launch' into the *5:2 Juice Diet*, here's the potential head start you can get:

> 'Feel great today, 6lbs down and reduced my body fat per cent by 3 per cent. Slept really well all week and no problems getting up in the morning. Going to carry on with the 5:2 Juice Diet. Thanks Jason.'
>
> — Suzanne

> 'Lost 7lbs and Hubbie lost 10lbs — we are both now Juicy Converts! Feeling so much healthier too!!'
>
> — Ellen W

> 'Love this book, I tried it for 5 days, lost 8lbs, skin healthier, more energy, no worries about what to eat, and NO MORE SLIMMING CLASSES, YIPPEE, I'M FREE.'
>
> — Marlene

'Excellent! I lost 8lb in 5 days, continued til day 8 and lost 10lb in total. I had more energy, I'm sleeping better too.'

— Sarah G

'I've done the 5 day plan 3 times over 4 weeks and lost 19.5lbs altogether!!! I'm a very happy customer.'

— Mrs P

I would deff recommend. I read the book first then used the app for shopping notes, videos and quick reminders.'

— Stella

'Started my juicing with the 5lbs in 5 Days — I have lost 10lbs! The results are incredible — 12st 2lbs on Monday morning, this morning (Saturday) 11st 6lbs. Amazing! Thank you Jason Vale, this just goes to show it truly does work!'

— Louise T

'Woohoo — finished 5 Days last night and down 11lbs on the scales this morning! Love juicing.'

— Rebecca H

'I lost 11.5 lbs and haven't had this much energy in a very long time! Also some of my Crohn's disease issues have subsided.'

— Christina S

'I cannot believe how easy it was. I never felt hungry and now feel fantastic and will continue to keep on juicing. I lost an amazing 13.5lbs in 5 days.'

— Janette W

'So impressed, my husband and I have just completed the 5lbs in 5 Days. I have lost 10.5 pounds and my husband has lost 7.5 pounds! I've had so many comments that I look fresh and slimmer. Thank you Jason!'

— Claire O

These are tiny snippets from the thousands of testimonials I have received over the years about the *5lbs in 5 Days* juice plan. Momentum is everything and nothing will convince you more of *why to* juice than getting those kind of results in such a short space of time. When you drop that kind of weight in such a short space of time, you're completely sold and moving to two days of juicing a week is a no brainer. I was speaking with a cab driver the other day about weight loss etc. (as this tends to happen when they ask what I do!) and he said that if he doesn't get significant results in the first week of a diet, he folds immediately. To put it not so delicately, his exact words were, 'They say if you lose a pound a week steadily that's better than dropping 10lbs in a week, but **** that, I can crap more than a pound!'

I will tell you now, if you decide to start with a five-day juicy bang, it will be the best decision you have ever made. You will not only 'jump the queue' up on the weight loss front, but you'll 100 per cent sold on this concept and you'll breeze into the *5:2 Juice Diet*. Once again though, this is only a suggestion, a *strong suggestion*, but just a suggestion. (Details of ways to do the five day 'juice fast' are found in 'The Q & A Session' (PAGE 219/CHAPTER 9). Please do not simply follow five of the 5:2 juice days which are laid out in this book, they are designed for a two-day a week *5:2 Juice Diet*, not a full five-day 'juice fast' – so please read the section in the Q & A if you choose to launch yourself into this).

If you're still not convinced by a full juice diet to launch your juicy 5:2 way of life, here's one last nudge. I have only added this in as, yesterday I met a family who I feel just may tip the balance if you're on the fence on this one. I met the Cunningham family at my filming studio as they had agreed to be on my YouTube show '*Juicing With Jason*'. I read their email only two weeks ago and, although we get hundreds every month, theirs stood out more than most. I thought I'd share it here:

'Juicing has transformed our lives. We have learned how to clean eat, how the body needs the right fuel & if you feed it right, then your body will take care of itself.

So we started on our juicy journey in May 2014. Our wedding anniversary was in April and Roy's sister asked what we would like for a present. We still don't really know why but Roy just said 'a juicer.' We subsequently received one which came with a book by Jason Vale in the book it mentioned a 3 day detox. For some unknown reason I just decided I wanted to do the 3 days. I'd never heard of Jason Vale so went home and googled him.

At the same time Roy had been quite poorly he'd had his knee replaced the year before and was struggling with the limitations this had brought him. He was being monitored for high blood pressure. As my carer, he'd been dealing with a lot including the loss of his Dad. So he wasn't sleeping well and seemed to be slipping into depression. The Dr had decided to put him on high blood pressure tablets. They sent him home to monitor his blood pressure for two weeks and then to return to the doctor for the dosage to be decided on.

Back to googling Jason Vale, I then discovered Jason Vale's 7lbs in 7 days book, app and I decided to do that instead of 3 days detox. Because of my dislike of any kind of diet, calorie counting etc. I decided to do this just for health benefits so I didn't weigh myself. Roy decided to join me with the boys just looking on mildly amused at these crazy parents. Well, we just felt so incredibly well and weight fell off us both. (Roy decided to give a healthy diet a chance and decided to not go back to the Dr until he had his diet under control.) As well as doing the 7 day detox: we were learning all about how the foods you eat affect you, not only physically but mentally too. Haydn then decided he wanted to do the 7 days, so over the space of 3 weeks we all completed the 7 day detox. We all felt so well I personally gained six hours in a day! I was used to waking up at 9am very sluggish and, as I'm recovering from post-traumatic stress disorder I would be so exhausted by 1pm I'd be asleep for 3 hrs. After juicing I was up at 6am doing a two-mile walk and didn't need a sleep in the afternoon. Honestly I felt like I had been given my life back. No longer was I just a robot dragging myself through each day. Now I had energy and amazingly the weight just fell off me.

Haydn was losing incredible amounts but we never weighed each week, only about once a month. We then moved on to the 14-days plan and had a juice meal. Roy and I have completed the 28-Day Super Juice Me. We have done 5-day as well. But mostly we have one juice a day with clean eating. There is nothing in our house that is processed. Before juicing our diet was 99 per cent ready meals now we have nothing processed. We do treat ourselves, we have a rule that a planned treat is OK but an unplanned one is not. This means we really think about what we want as a treat and it's amazing how often if you really think about it, you decide you don't really want it in the first place. It also means the Boys are always saying 'Mum, I'm having a planned treat right now'. THANK YOU Jason, you have managed to build a clear path through all the dietary confusion out there. You speak a language that all can understand. You take quite deep points and portray them in a way all can understand. You have touched our family's lives and given us a very precious second chance to eat well and live life to the full.'

— Cherry Cunningham

When interviewing them on the show, Cherry Cunnigham (the mother) mentioned she now adheres to the *5:2 Juice Diet* principles. Cherry, Roy and Haydn have dropped a colossal 17 stone (238lbs) between them in just one year. This is the power of *consistent commitment* and was made possible by an initial seven-day full-on 'juice fast'. It was this 'juice convincer' which ultimately led to the incredible success the whole family are experiencing now. Not only have they dropped an incredible amount of weight, but Roy's blood pressure is now normal and Cherry has gained six hours in a day, that's ten years! This family have said it was the results they got in such a short space of time that led them to eating well and adopting a *5:2 Juice Diet* way of life. This is why I wanted to add their story here, as a final attempt to nudge you in that direction. Again, it is not imperative to do a full 'juice fast' first and the *5:2 Juice Diet* as a stand alone, I just want you to get the results you are ultimately looking for and, after 15 years of doing this, I know how people tick when it comes to weight loss and health. However, even if you choose to simply go *5:2 Juice Diet* and skip the 'juice launch' into it, you will be miles ahead of most people and you will still get extremely good results.

You should by now have a strong enough *why* to at least try this on for size. When I say 'try it on for size', I don't mean just do two days of juicing one week and then throw in the towel, I mean commit to at least a month of this *5:2 Juice Diet System*. Juicing for just two days and then never again won't do anything for you in the long-term and won't convince you of anything, you need to experience this *5:2 Juice System* for at least a month. If you're not convinced by then, and haven't had any results, then throw in the juice towel, but at least give it a shot. I mean, you've read this far into the book, now take that all-important next step, the one that many who read a book of this nature seem to not manage:

TAKE ACTION!

It still baffles me that, even after someone invests in a book like this *and* takes the time to read it, some fail to take action and still order a pizza! You have picked up this book because you want to make a lasting change in the area of weight loss and health, you've come this far, so now do whatever it takes to do it.

Many of you will already be sold on the idea and simply itching to get started. If that's you, I'll be getting to the full *5:2 Juice Diet* plan very soon, but the key behind anything involving *consistent commitment* is finding ways to make it easy. If something proves just a little too much for us, we often give up, so on that note here are your...

TOP TEN TIPS

FOR MAKING IT EASY!

4

1. WATCH SUPER JUICE ME! THE BIG JUICE EXPERIMENT

Perspective is *everything* and nothing will give you more perspective, before starting the *5:2 Juice Diet*, than watching the ground-breaking health documentary, *Super Juice Me! The Big Juice Experiment.* This is where I took eight people with 22 different health conditions between them and put them on nothing but juice for 28 days at my health retreat in Portugal. In my opinion, nothing will convince you of the health and weight loss benefits of juicing more than this film. Seriously, if you're still looking for a *why*, then watch it! In terms of perspective, there's nothing like watching people who did 28 days straight on juice alone. To watch the film for FREE go to *www.superjuiceme.com* or, by the time this book is released, it should be on other platforms. The film is not only educational, but also extremely moving and incredibly inspirational. It not only has the potential to get you inspired to do the *5:2 Juice Challenge*, but you may even kick off your juicy life with the full five-day programme I *strongly* advised. For those with extreme health and weight issues to overcome, it may even inspire you to really kick off with the biggest juicy bang of all – the full *Super Juice Me! 28-Day Juice Plan*, followed by this *5:2 Juice Diet*.

2. GET THE RIGHT EQUIPMENT!

As with most things in life, you need the right tools for the job in hand, and juicing is no exception to that rule. Nothing will put you off juicing faster than having the wrong juicer, so you need to get this right from the start. The right juicer for you may not be the right juicer for someone else. Please make a point of reading 'So What Juicer Is Best, Jase?' (PAGE 239/CHAPTER 10) to get a very clear picture of what juicer *you* will need. You want to make this as easy as possible and the last thing you want on your maiden voyage is a juicer that doesn't fit with *you*. The wrong decision here could put a solid nail in your juicing coffin for now and ever more – so please read that section.

3. MAKE YOUR JUICES IN ADVANCE!

Freshly made and consumed within one hour of making will always be the best way, if that fits in with your lifestyle. The minute freshly extracted juice is exposed to air, it starts to oxidize and nutrients begin to be lost. Having said that, very rarely does this model fit into the average person's hectic life. Not only that, but most people really don't want to wash their juicer four times a day. With this in mind there are a couple of options to make life easier:

A. Make all the juices for the day, put them into flasks, dark bottles or 'boosters'. Keep them as cold as possible and don't allow oxygen or light in. These will keep nicely for the day.

B. Make all the juices the night before the two-day 'fast', put the first two in flasks for the morning of day one and simply freeze the rest. You can then remove the afternoon juices for day one in the morning, put them in the fridge and, by the afternoon, they should be ready to drink. That night, remove the frozen juices for day two, place into the fridge and they'll be ready the next day. Unlike cooking, freezing preserves the nutrients so hardly anything is lost. If you have ever used our Juice Master Delivered service *www.juicemasterdelivered.com* (where we make all the juices for you and deliver them frozen to your home), you'll have noticed that all the bottles aren't see through. This is deliberate, as we don't want any light going in. If you have used this service, you'll know that you can always wash the bottles and use these for freezing when making your own juices.

C. Make all your juices in a slow 'cold press'

juicer. The slower the juicer the less heat friction applied and the longer your juice will keep. This type of juicer is becoming more and more popular as people become much more aware of the different types of juicers and what they do. The best result, other than making them 100 per cent fresh and drinking within the hour, would be to make them in a 'cold press' juicer and then freeze. I am however aware that the vast majority of people have 'fast' juicers (and often for good 'I just need to juice and go' reasons) and juicing in this type of juicer and freezing is still great! For more see 'What Juicer Is Best, Jase?' PAGE 239.

4. LITTLE TIP FOR NOT HAVING TO CLEAN YOUR JUICER FOUR TIMES DAY!

If you don't want to make your juices in advance and freeze them all, but instead want to make them fresh each time, then here's a little tip. If you have room and are in a household where you are able to, for the two 'juice fast' days, take out the upper shelves of your fridge and leave enough space where your juicer will fit (clearly this all depends on the size of your juicer and size of your fridge). You then make your juice and 'rinse' your juicer immediately afterwards without taking it apart. This is done by placing an empty jug under the juice spout, turning on the juicer and pouring warm water into it. This won't 'clean' your juicer, but it will 'rinse it'. If you have a Retro Cold Press juicer it has actually been designed with this 'rinsing' in mind, but the same principle can be applied to any juicer with lesser effect. You then place the whole juicer into your fridge to stop any fruit flies and so on getting to the machine. You then pop it into your fridge until the next time you make a juice. You do this until your final juice, after which you clean the juicer properly. The only other thing you may need to do between 'rinses' is remove the lid of the juicer and take out any excess pulp (which might be clogging the machine and causing 'bits' in the juice.) This is still a lot easier than actually cleaning the juicer. You may also need to empty the actual pulp container. This is a nice compromise and guarantees the healthiest juice as it is fresh every time. If the juicer cannot fit into the fridge, for whatever reason, then some people leave it out on the work surface, 'rinse' it and cover it with a tea towel or similar.

5. KEEP YOUR JUICER ON SHOW!

No matter how small your kitchen, make a permanent space for your juicer. When I set out to 'Juice The World', my mission was to make a juicer and blender as common as a kettle and toaster in everyone's kitchen. Like the kettle and toaster, it should take pride of place. The reason why the bread maker, steamer, rice cooker and so on are all in darkness in a cupboard, is because we don't use them everyday, but your juicer and blender are tools I am hoping you will use daily. You are much more likely to use them daily if they are out in the open, armed and ready for use. You may think you don't have room for such items in a room where there's a constant battle for space on the worktop, but this is important. We need the right fuel going into us daily and it's part of your fuel station and should take pride of place. If you are really struggling for space, get your microwave and throw it out the window, that will free up a nice amount of space! (I am joking clearly before some numpty actually throws it out of the window!)

6. DRINK, DRINK, DRINK!

Even though you are having nothing but liquid nutrition, in order to make your 'juice fast' days easier, I advise you use water and herbal teas as a tool for curbing any hunger. Hunger pangs come and go, and usually within a very short space of time, but if you do feel the need to take something on board, then water and herbal teas will become your best friends. Personally, I love fresh mint tea and a large cup of that usually fills any hunger void I may be feeling at that time. If you are out and about, all the major coffee chains now do excellent herbal and green teas. If I'm in Starbucks, for example, on a 'fast day' I'll grab a Vente (that's large to you and me) peppermint tea with two teabags. What's great is a) it's SO much cheaper than a milky hot shake (otherwise known as a latte) and you get served straight away, no waiting down the end of the counter for your name to be called. Keeping a bottle of water with you at all times is also a great tool, add lemon or lime to make it slightly more interesting.

7. GET FRUITY WHEN YOU NEED TO!

If you really feel you need to eat something, or you are in a position where you cannot use your juicer, let fruit be thy juice. All fruits are over 85 per cent pure organic liquid nutrition and have been, by their very nature, pre-digested by the plant. This means fruit requires very little digestion from us and is easily absorbed and utilised. Remember, the reason for juicing is to get raw *vegetables* into us in the easiest and most bioavailable way. The nutrients in raw fruits on the other hand, tend to be readily bio-available and easily digested. This is why many fruits are great for 'fasting days' if you cannot get a juice, or you simply have an overwhelming desire to use your teeth. A banana usually does wonders and, at only 100 calories and loaded with essential nutrients, they really are the best 'juice on the go'. Bananas are over 85 per cent water, despite looking solid, they are extremely easily digested and perfect for when out and about. Watermelon is another wonderful fruit and is 99 per cent water and as good as a juice. I often use watermelon when on 'juice days' as a slice of watermelon is effectively pure juice in a solid form. Watermelon is also loaded with essential minerals, such as zinc and selenium, making them exceptionally good for the skin. Oranges are also great, along with pears, apples and so on. They are pure juice, contained within fibre, that the body has no difficulty extracting once consumed. The other fruit that can really help any 'juice fast' day is the king of all fruits, and could be argued the king of all foods – avocado. The humble avocado has got me out of hunger trouble a few times, this is because the incredible amount of good fat it contains is perfect for regulating appetite. I either simply skip a juice and eat an avocado instead (usually my evening one), or I add half an avocado to a juice if I am particularly hungry. You will need to 'blend' the avocado with the juice as avocados are too much of a complex fat and don't juice, despite being over 85 per cent water. When I do eat the avocado, I don't just wolf it down, I pick a nice large, ripe one, cut it in half, remove the stone, add some lemon juice and cracked black pepper and eat straight from 'nature's bowl'. This is why I never understand when someone says it's hard to find a healthy snack! Ideally, you will stick to the juices on your two 'juice fast' days, but if it's going to be a case of falling down altogether or having an avocado or banana, have the fruit! It's not always practical to juice either and this is why you should always get fruity when you need to on 'juice fast' days.

8. MAKE YOUR WEEKEND YOUR 'HUMAN DAYS'

Clearly it's your call what days you do what, but most choose to make the weekends their 'human days'. The weekends tend to be the days we socialise more than the others and it means we don't alienate ourselves. You can of course choose any two days as your 'human days' or not have any 'human days', as not everyone feels they need it, but I have found as most socialising takes place during the weekend, that's the best time to allocate for these days.

9. STAY JUICED ALL WEEK!

Although this is a *5:2 Juice Diet* where you will be juicing for just two days a week, I *strongly* advise you keep in the habit of having juice for breakfast for a least three of the other five days a week. Juicing then becomes a habit and ultimately makes the two 'juice fast' days easier. This is your call clearly, but this is a great habit to get into for many reasons. I have mapped out 'A Rough Week In The Life...' (PAGE 209/CHAPTER 8) to give you an idea of what I mean and how it should work.

10. BRING IT TO LIFE — GET THE APP!

The *5:2 Juice Diet* app came out long before the book and when it was first launched, it had just two weeks worth of recipes in it and no videos of me making the recipes. The app was cheap at just over £2, but because people were used to my apps showing how to make the recipes, some felt they had been short-changed. It is interesting that people will pay £3 for a coffee and yet think £2 on an app with a solid, nutritionally sound plan is too much, but that is the world we live in today. Because people wanted the recipes brought to life, I have done just that. In the new version of the app I bring a few of the recipes to life á la Jamie Oliver style and give a few 5:2 tips. The app is not an essential at all, but simply an additional tool to make the 5:2 juicy life a little easier and to connect with someone on screen so you don't feel you're alone in this! The app also helps a great deal with shopping, as there's an interactive shopping list that automatically generates a list of whatever 'week' you have chosen. You will see when you get to the plan, that I have created 32 recipes, which actually add up to four weeks worth, as you'll be having four a day for two days a week. If you want to 'mix and match' then the auto generator on the app will work it out for you. I have, of course, added a 'per week' shopping list to this book, but if you're shaking it up, then the app works well for this.

HOW TO 5:2 JUICE DIET

THE SYSTEM

5

The *5:2 Juice Diet* principles are, as already mentioned, extremely simple:

1. **You consume four '125/150'calorie juices a day for two days a week.**

2. **You eat 'clean' for three days a week.**

3. **You have two 'Human Days' a week.**

You may choose to follow the *5:2 Juice Diet* or, what I describe as my *5:2 Juice Diet System*. When following the *5:2 Juice Diet* you will consume four 125/150 calorie juices per day for two days a week and eat whatever floats your boat for the other five days. However I am hoping that after reading this book you will be following the *5:2 Juice Diet System*, which incorporates principles two and three above. Funnily enough, many people who kick off with the recommended full-on five day 'juice fast' and then follow it with the *5:2 Juice System*, choose not only to eat well for just three days a week, but don't even take the 'human day' option! However, the key principle is to commit to two full days of juicing every week forever more. Even if you fall slightly by the wayside and your three 'clean eating' days turn into *no* 'clean eating' days, you'll still be getting an enormous amount of nutrition on your two 'juice fast' days.

To sum up, do what works for you and your lifestyle, but at a minimum follow principle one and live for two days a week on freshly extracted juice.

NO NEED TO COUNT CALORIES

The good news is that unlike the '*5:2 Food Diet*', you won't need to count calories or start weighing and measuring anything as I've done all of that for you. All you have to do is make the recipes and drink them at the times suggested. Each recipe is between 125/150 calories and conforms to the original *5:2 Diet* principles.

TAKE THE FOUR WEEK

5:2 JUICE CHALLENGE

The idea is for the *5:2 Juice Diet* to become a way of life, for life. However, the thought of committing to anything for life can be daunting for some, especially if you are still unsure about juicing at this stage. This is why I encourage you to commit to at least four weeks, that way you give yourself a fighting chance of creating a *5:2 Juice Diet* habit for life. I have created 32 delicious 5:2 'calorie controlled' juices – one month's worth. More importantly I have made sure there is plenty of variety for each week, as if they were all the same every week for the rest of your life; you'd soon get very bored! I encourage you to follow the first four weeks to the letter to see which ones you like and which ones you'll end up leaving out. Having said that, if you see a recipe you know won't work for you for whatever reason, such as being allergic or you know you hate a certain ingredient, then clearly feel free to choose a recipe from a different week, but as previously mentioned, I do encourage you to follow the four week *5:2 Juice Diet* plan as laid out. It will also mean you don't have to think about what you have, plus the shopping list for each week has all been worked out for you too. At the end of the four-week challenge, you can then pick which week's recipes worked best for you in terms of taste and stick with those from that point. If you have the *5:2 Juice Diet* app then it automatically works out the shopping list from the recipes you choose, but if you don't have the app then good old-fashioned pen, paper and a calculator will do the trick!

RECIPE IDEAS FOR THE
5:2 JUICE DIET SYSTEM

I mentioned earlier that I'd be giving you some recipe ideas for when you are 'eating clean' for at least three of the five non-juice days. I also mentioned I'd give a 'week in the life of the *5:2 Juice Diet System'* to give you a rough idea of what your week may look like. Both of these you will find *after* I have mapped out the 'Four Week 5:2 Juice Challenge' (PAGE 186/SUPER FAST FOOD and PAGE 209 /CHAPTER 8). I would like to remind you to make a point of reading 'The Q & A Session' (PAGE 219 /CHAPTER 9) it will answer all of your burning 'yeah but… ' questions. Right, I think it's time to crack on and get straight into…

FOUR WEEK

5:2

JUICE

CHALLENGE

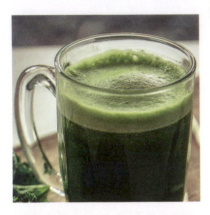
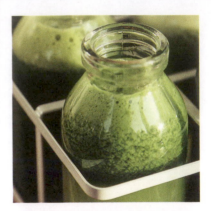
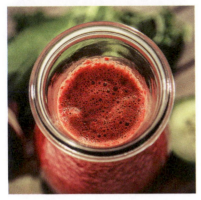
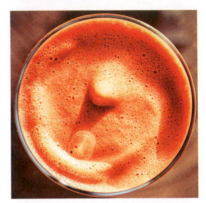
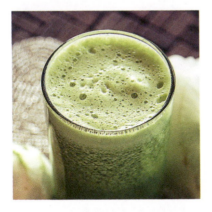
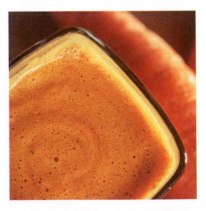
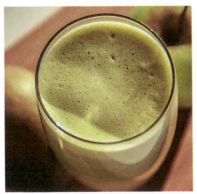
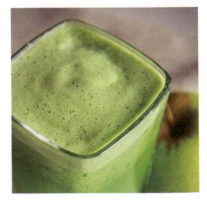

W E E K

O N E

THE JUICES

DAY ONE

9am	POWER PLANT
1pm	VIVA LA VEGGIE
4pm	FENNEL FURY
7pm	PEARFECTION

DAY TWO

9am	CLEAN 'N' GREEN
1pm	BASIL BLUSH
4pm	GINGER NINJA
7pm	FRESH 'N' WILD

SHOPPING LIST

Apples (Golden Delicious or Gala)	9	Pears	3
Raw Beetroots (small)	2	Pineapple (medium)	1
Broccoli Stem (or use florets)	7cm	Spinach Leaves	175g
Carrots (medium)	4	Fresh Basil	12g
Celery Stalks	5	Fennel (small)	1 bulb
Courgette/Zucchini (medium)	1	Raw Ginger	80g
Cucumbers (medium)	2	Fresh Mint	6g
Kale	60g		
Lemon (unwaxed)	1		
Limes (unwaxed)	2		
Living Salad	1 pot		
Mango (ripe)	1		
Orange	1		
Parsnip (medium)	1		

KEEP IT IN THE FAMILY!

Broccoli is a cruciferous

vegetable and part of the

Brassicaceae family along with

cabbage, cauliflower, bok choi

and brussels sprouts.

POWER PLANT

The power of Mother Nature really goes to work in this juice. Chlorophyll rich leafy greens, an undertone of cucumber, celery, broccoli and the bitter sweet creaminess of pineapple and lime.

INGREDIENTS:

Pineapple ½ (peeled)
Cucumber ¼
Lime ½ (peeled, white pith left on)
Celery 1 ½ stalks
Spinach Leaves 1 large handful
Broccoli Stem 2.5 cm (or use florets)
Ice 1 small handful

INSTRUCTIONS:

Juice all the ingredients.

Once you've finished, pour over ice and enjoy.

JUICING TIP:

If you are using a fast (centrifugal) juicer always remember to tightly pack the spinach in between the harder produce to ensure maximum juice extraction.

However, if you are using a slow (masticating/cold press) juicer then feel free to juice in any order you fancy as these machines are designed to handle leafy greens.

SO WHAT IS IN THIS BABY?

This beautiful green blend is packed with sunlight energy and contains a wealth of vitamins, minerals, amino acids and enzymes.

Celery and Cucumber provide the perfect balance of sodium and potassium which works like a natural electrolyte, great for pre and post workouts to reduce achy muscles and replace lost salts.

Pineapple contains bromelain, an enzyme effective in reducing inflammation, which may help people suffering with arthritis or joint pain. Bromelain also dissolves mucus, so helpful in reducing the symptoms of hay fever and asthma. Spinach is wonderfully rich in manganese, magnesium and iron as well as key vitamins such as A, C and K.

SMALL & TASTY

Courgettes are best picked
when they are smaller as
this is when they are at their
most flavoursome.

VIVA LA VEGGIE

Sweet meets savoury in this nutritionally
fuelled veggie deluxe meal in a glass.

INGREDIENTS:

Apples 2
Carrot 1
Celery 1 stalk
Spinach Leaves 1 handful
Kale 1 handful
Cucumber ¼
Broccoli Stem 2.5 cm (or use florets)
Raw Beetroot 1
Courgette/Zucchini ¼
Ice 1 small handful

INSTRUCTIONS:

Juice all the ingredients.

Pour over ice and enjoy.

JUICING TIP:

If you are using a fast (centrifugal) juicer always
remember to tightly pack the spinach and kale in
between the harder produce to ensure maximum
juice extraction.

However, if you are using a slow (masticating/cold
press) juicer then feel free to juice in any order you
fancy as these machines are designed to handle leafy
greens.

SO WHAT IS IN THIS BABY?

This viva la vegetable medley, with a hint of sweetness, is packed with chlorophyll. Chlorophyll is
formed in the cells of plant leaves and is what gives leafy greens their green colour.

This tasty juice is an excellent immune booster; rich in vitamin A which helps to maintain healthy,
vibrant skin, strong bones and bright eyes. It's also fuelled with minerals such as chlorine,
manganese, calcium, iron, sodium, phosphorus, potassium, copper, chromium and magnesium.
Minerals are essential for so many important functions in the body, including strong bone growth
and, most importantly, turning our food into energy.

FENNELING GOOD!

Fennel has been said to
help release endorphins
into the bloodstream.
These 'feel good' chemicals
help to heighten your mood.

FENNEL FURY

The mighty fusion of deep leafy greens, sweet apple and lime beautifully compliments the warming undertone of ginger and the natural aniseed notes of fennel.

INGREDIENTS:

Apple 1
Fennel 1 bulb
Spinach Leaves 1 small handful
Kale 1 small handful
Lime 1 (peeled, white pith left on)
Raw Ginger 2.5 cm
Ice 1 small handful

INSTRUCTIONS:

Juice all the ingredients.

Pour over ice and enjoy.

JUICING TIP:

If you are using a fast (centrifugal) juicer always remember to tightly pack the spinach and kale in between the harder produce to ensure maximum juice extraction.

However, if you are using a slow (masticating/cold press) juicer then feel free to juice in any order you fancy as these machines are designed to handle leafy greens.

SO WHAT IS IN THIS BABY?

This mineral rich meal in a glass contains calcium, chromium, cobalt, iron, magnesium, manganese, phosphorus, potassium, selenium, silicon, sodium and zinc.

Fennel contains quercetin, a flavonoid that has been shown to have excellent anti-inflammatory properties. It is also high in vitamin C and heart-friendly potassium. Fennel is an excellent source of antioxidant vitamins A, C, and K. The anethole found in fennel has been found to have antibacterial and anti-fungal properties.

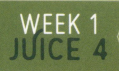

AS SWEET AS SUGAR

Did you know that, before
the sugar beet industry was
established in the 19th century,
parsnips were commonly used
as a sweetener?

PEARFECTION

A subtle base of sweet apple, ripened pears and thick, creamy parsnip juice; combined with a fresh mint breeze, the coolness of cucumber and a twist of lime.

INGREDIENTS:

Apple 1
Pears 2
Parsnip 1
Cucumber ¼
Lime ½ (peeled, white pith left on)
Fresh Mint 1 small handful
Ice 1 small handful

INSTRUCTIONS:

Juice all the ingredients.

Simply pour over ice and enjoy.

JUICING TIP:

If you are using a fast (centrifugal) juicer always remember to tightly pack the mint in between the harder produce to ensure maximum juice extraction.

However, if you are using a slow (masticating/cold press) juicer then feel free to juice in any order you fancy as these machines are designed to handle leafy greens.

SO WHAT IS IN THIS BABY?

Pears are one of the highest fibre fruits. Their juice is loaded with pectin, a soluble fibre that acts like a gel in the intestine to help sweep through waste and trap any toxins that may be lurking.

Parsnips are a great source of vitamins C, K, E and folic acid. They also contain many important minerals including iron, calcium, manganese, copper and potassium.

Cooling cucumber juice is rich in vitamins A, B, C, beta carotene, K and folic acid and a wealth of minerals including sodium, potassium, calcium and phosphorus. Cucumbers are also rich in silicon and sulphur, which stimulate the kidneys to flush away toxins.

RIPEN YOUR MANGO
You can speed up the ripening process by putting mangos into a paper bag at room temperature.

CLEAN 'N' GREEN

A fresh and fruity green blend but not as we know it! I've added in the tantalizingly tropical taste of mouthwatering mango to sweeten this baby up and turning this 'Clean 'n' Green into something truly supreme!

INGREDIENTS:

Apple 1
Mango ½ (ripe)
Broccoli Stem 2.5 cm (or use florets)
Celery ½ stalk
Cucumber ¼
Spinach Leaves 1 handful
Kale 1 handful
Raw Ginger 1 cm
Ice 1 small handful

INSTRUCTIONS:

Juice all the ingredients.

Pour over ice in your favourite glass and enjoy.

JUICING TIP:

If you are using a fast (centrifugal) juicer always remember to tightly pack any leafy greens and the mango in between the harder produce to ensure maximum juice extraction.

However, if you are using a slow (masticating/cold press) juicer then feel free to juice in any order you fancy as these machines are designed to handle leafy greens and soft fruit.

SO WHAT IS IN THIS BABY?

Sweet and juicy mangos are a good source of vitamins A, C and E as well as phosphorus, potassium and magnesium. Vitamin E is a powerful antioxidant and fat-soluble vitamin that is important for promoting healthy, glowing skin.

MANGO TIP:

To easily remove the large flat 'stone' place the mango on its side and cut it slightly off centre so you miss the stone as you cut through. Take the mango half and 'score' into cubes, turn the mango inside out and cut the pieces from the skin. Repeat on the other side. The mango will produce a very thick but extremely nutritious and sweet juice, which balances the bitterness of the greens beautifully.

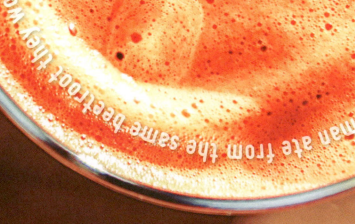

BLUSHING BEETROOT   In days of old many cultures believed that if a man and a woman ate from the same beetroot they would fall in love.

BASIL BLUSH—BOOM! BOOM!

Fresh, fragrant and bursting with a certain je ne sais quoi. This juice mixes earthy notes from the finest root vegetables with the juiciest apples and pears and the soothing sweet-scent of basil and ginger to create this ruby red, cheek warmer!

INGREDIENTS:

Apple 1
Pear 1
Carrot 1
Raw Beetroot ½
Fresh Basil 1 small handful
Raw Ginger 1cm
Ice 1 small handful

INSTRUCTIONS:

Juice all the ingredients.

Pour over ice and enjoy.

JUICING TIP:

If you are using a fast (centrifugal) juicer always remember to tightly pack the basil in between the harder produce to ensure maximum juice extraction.

However, if you are using a slow (masticating/cold press) juicer then feel free to juice in any order you fancy as these machines are designed to handle leafy greens.

SO WHAT IS IN THIS BABY?

As well as helping to create a fragrant and delicious juice, basil also raises the nutritional game. It is a great source of vitamin K, an essential vitamin for blood clotting and healing cuts and grazes.

Fresh Basil leaves are also an excellent source of iron, which is responsible for producing red blood cells that then carry oxygen around the body. This juice is also loaded with vitamins B, C, beta-carotene as well as sodium, magnesium, potassium and calcium.

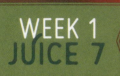

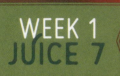

WEEK 1
JUICE 7

LEMONY FRESH
Lemon is naturally anti-fungal
and antibacterial and is used
in many cleaning products.

GINJA NINJA

'King Carrot' takes on the crispness of the mighty apple, whilst celery and zesty lemon join forces to embrace the final pungent kick of ginger. This is definitely a juice not to be messed with!

INGREDIENTS:

Apples 2
Carrots 2
Celery 1 stick
Lemon 2.5 cm slice (wax free, rind on)
Raw Ginger 1 cm
Ice 1 small handful

INSTRUCTIONS:

Simply juice the lot in whatever order you fancy!

Once done, pour over ice and enjoy.

SO WHAT IS IN THIS BABY?

Carrots boost our intake of the antioxidant vitamins C and E. These nutrients prevent cell damage caused by free radicals and help to maintain cell structure. Carrots boast a whole host of B vitamins, which can help to alleviate feelings of tiredness and fatigue.

Ginger is often referred to as being a root but it's actually an underground stem called a rhizome. Ginger improves the absorption of essential nutrients in the body. Gingerols are the potent anti-inflammatory compounds found in ginger and appear to reduce pain and improve mobility.

LIVE A LITTLE LONGER

'Living salad' leaves are fresher and
can last longer than those in bags
because they are still in the soil.

FRESH 'N' WILD

The freshness of cucumber and celery, the wildness of green leaves straight from the earth and a hint of sunshine citrus and ginger. This juice will definitely take your taste buds on an adventure to remember!

INGREDIENTS:

Apple 1
Orange 1 (peeled, white pith left on)
Living Salad 1 pot
Lemon 2.5 cm slice (wax free, rind on)
Cucumber ¼
Celery 1 stick
Raw Ginger 2.5 cm
Ice 1 small handful

INSTRUCTIONS:

Juice all the ingredients.

Pour over ice and enjoy.

JUICING TIP:

If you are using a fast (centrifugal) juicer always remember to tightly pack any leafy greens in between the harder produce to ensure maximum juice extraction.

However, if you are using a slow (masticating/cold press) juicer then feel free to juice in any order you fancy as these machines are designed to handle leafy greens.

SO WHAT IS IN THIS BABY?

Vitamins A, C, E, K and those all-important complex B vitamins all feature in this juice. It also has iron, calcium, potassium, magnesium, phosphorus, selenium and that's only naming a few!

LIVING SALAD

Most super markets sell a 'living salad' of some kind. They are called 'living' salads because they are still in the soil and still very much 'living'. If you can't find them in the supermarket, at your local farmer's market or you don't grown your own, then simply use spinach (or if you're feeling brave you could try nettle instead!). I am just trying to add the 'wild' element to this 'Fresh 'n' Wild recipe.

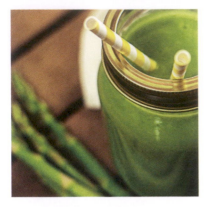
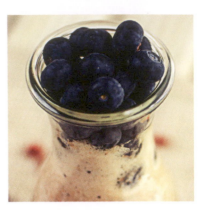
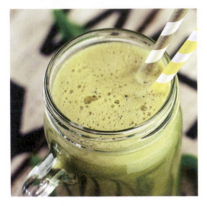
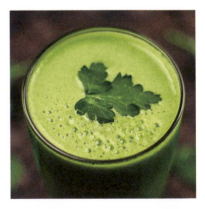

W E E E K

T W O

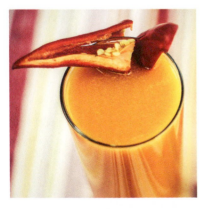
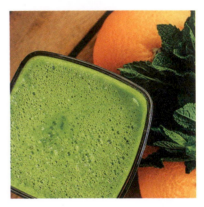
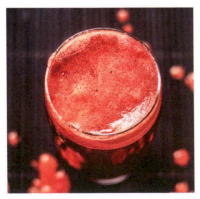
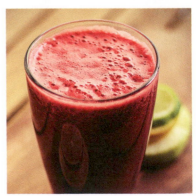

THE JUICES

DAY ONE

9am   ASPARAGUS, PEAR & AVOCADO BLEND

1pm   APPLE, PEAR, MINT INFUSION

4pm   THAI SPICE SUPER JUICE

7pm   ROOT OF ALL GOOD

DAY TWO

9am   GOGI, BLUEBERRY & COCONUT POWER BLEND

1pm   ORANGE, MINT & SPINACH INFUSION

4pm   PARSLEY LEMON HEALTH HITTER

7pm   SWEET + SOUR SENSATION

SHOPPING LIST

Apples (Golden Delicious or Gala)	6	Parsnip (medium)		1
Asparagus Spears	2	Pears		5
Avocado (ripe)	1	Pineapple (medium)		1
Banana (ripe and fair-trade)	1	Spinach Leaves		85g
Raw Beetroots (small)	2	Strawberries (fresh or frozen)		30g
Blueberries	20g	Coconut Water		350ml
Carrots (medium)	2	Raw Ginger		90g
Red Chilli	1	Fresh Mint		25g
Cucumber (medium)	2	Fresh Parsley		20g
Goji Berries	10g			
Lemon (unwaxed)	1			
Limes (unwaxed)	3			
Mango (ripe)	1			
Orange	1			

PERFECTLY RIPE!

Pop off the stem at the top of your avocado, if it comes away easily and it's green underneath it's ripe and ready to eat.

ASPARAGUS, PEAR & AVOCADO BLEND

Rich, creamy, thick and incredibly filling — exactly what you want when doing the 5:2 Juice Diet.

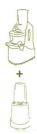

INGREDIENTS:

Apple 1

Pears 2

Cucumber ¼

Asparagus 2 spears

Avocado ¼ (ripe)

Ice 1 small handful

INSTRUCTIONS:

Juice the cucumber, asparagus, pears and apple.

Scoop the flesh from the avocado into your blender. Add a little ice and whiz until creamy.

Pour into a glass of your fancy and sip slowly.

SO WHAT IS IN THIS BABY?

The natural fat from the avocado helps to regulate your appetite, lifts the sweet flavours of freshly extracted apple and pear juice. The cucumber adds freshness to the whole blend whilst the asparagus gives something extra on the nutritional front. All in all, an extremely powerful blend that will hit the mark every time.

Asparagus is low in calories and is very low in sodium. It is a good source of vitamin B, calcium, magnesium and zinc and a very good source of dietary fibre, protein, beta-carotene, vitamin C, vitamin E, vitamin K, thiamine and riboflavin.

A typical serving of avocado (100g) is said to be moderate to rich in several B vitamins and vitamin K, with good content of vitamin C, vitamin E and potassium.

YOU BUTTER BELIEVE IT

Pears were given the nickname
'butter fruit' in the 1700s

because of their soft

and buttery texture.

APPLE, PEAR & MINT INFUSION

Combine any fruit or vegetable juice with apple, pear and cucumber and
you'll always be onto a winner on both the taste and nutrition front
and the addition of fresh mint lifts this juice beautifully.

INGREDIENTS:

Apple 1
Pear 1
Cucumber ¼
Fresh Mint 1 small handful
Ice 1 small handful

INSTRUCTIONS:

Simply juice the lot and pour over ice.

JUICING TIP:

If you are using a fast (centrifugal) juicer always
remember to tightly pack the mint in between the
harder produce to ensure maximum juice extraction.

However, if you are using a slow (masticating/cold
press) juicer then feel free to juice in any order you
fancy as these machines are designed to handle leafy
greens.

SO WHAT IS IN THIS BABY?

This juice is not only loaded with soluble fibre to help 'keep everything moving' but it's a natural
diuretic, which will also help in the same direction.

Pears are a very good source of dietary fiber and a good source of copper, vitamin C and vitamin
K. Pears are also a concentrated source of phenolic phytonutrients including antioxidants and
anti-inflammatory flavonoids.

Fresh Mint leaves provide a considerable amount of vitamin A, as well as small amounts of
other vitamins such as vitamin C and B-complex vitamins. Vitamin A promotes healthy skin and
supports your immune system, which also helps cells to reproduce normally.

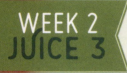

FEELING HOT! HOT! HOT!

Chillies burn the mouth due to alkaloid compounds, capsaicin, capsorubin and capsanthin.

THAI SUPER SPICE JUICE

The creamy sweetness of freshly extracted pineapple juice is
given a jolt with the inclusion of fiery hot chilli and ginger juice.

INGREDIENTS:

Apple 1
Pineapple ½ (peeled)
Mango ½ (ripe)
Lime 1 (peeled, white pith left on)
Red Chilli ½ (seeds removed)
Raw Ginger 3 cm
Ice 1 small handful

INSTRUCTIONS:

Juice the lot and pour over ice. Kick back, imagine
yourself on a sun-kissed beach in Thailand and enjoy!

JUICING TIP:

If you are using a fast (centrifugal) juicer always
remember to tightly pack the mango and chilli in
between the harder produce to ensure maximum juice
extraction.

However, if you are using a slow (masticating/cold
press) juicer then feel free to juice in any order you
fancy as these machines are designed to handle soft
fruits.

SO WHAT IS IN THIS BABY?

The fresh apple, rich mango and lime subtly calm the whole thing down, but not by too much, so
expect this bad boy to still pack one hell of a punch!

Nutritionally chillies are very high in potassium, magnesium and iron. Their very high vitamin C
content can also substantially increase the uptake of non-hermetic iron (all iron found in plants)
from other ingredients in a meal, such as beans and grains.

MANGO TIP:

To easily remove the large flat 'stone' place the mango on its side and cut it slightly off centre
so you miss the stone as you cut through. Take the mango half and 'score' into cubes, turn the
mango inside out and cut the pieces from the skin. Repeat on the other side.

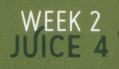

ROOTY TOOTY

Because root vegetables grow in the earth, they absorb a great deal of nutrients from the soil.

ROOT OF ALL GOOD

This recipe is aptly named as A) all of the ingredients have a root at their very core and B) because it's all good!

INGREDIENTS:

Raw Beetroot 1
Carrots 2
Parsnip 1
Raw Ginger 3 cm

INSTRUCTIONS:

There is no need to peel any of the ingredients, simply juice the lot, pour over ice, and imagine pottering around on a little allotment, and collecting up all of your home grown veggies in the sunshine.

Pour over ice and enjoy.

SO WHAT IS IN THIS BABY?

The sweetness (for a change) doesn't come from the inclusion of apple or pear but rather from the rich, sweet and freshly extracted juice from the humble carrot.

Carrots are a rich source of mineral salts such as potassium, cobalt, iron, magnesium, copper and phosphorus.

Beetroot juice is also surprisingly sweet, helping to mask the earthiness of this juice. Beetroot is renowned for cleansing the liver and the blood and is one of the most tested and proven vegetables for reducing blood pressure.

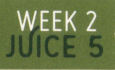

WASH & GO

Only wash your blueberries
just before eating them or
they will spoil more quickly.

GOGI BERRY, BLUEBERRY & COCONUT POWER BLEND

Coconut water, blended with the sweet, delicious, nutrient packed super berries that are 'goji' and 'blue', combine to make one of the highest antioxidant and mouth-watering blends on this plan.

INGREDIENTS:

Goji Berries 10 g
Blueberries 20 g
Coconut Water 350 ml
Banana ¼ (ripe)
Ice 1 small handful

INSTRUCTIONS:

No juicer is needed for this beauty, just its sidekick the blender.

Simply place all ingredients into the blender, whiz until smooth, pour into a glass over ice and sip slowly (you'll want to make this one last!).

SO WHAT IS IN THIS BABY?

Fresh coconut water contains a very good source of B-complex vitamins, vitamin C and a very substantial amount of the electrolyte potassium, as well as sodium. Together, these electrolytes help replenish electrolyte deficiency in the body. Coconut water also has a good composition of minerals such as calcium, iron, magnesium and zinc.

The addition of the creamy banana, adds plenty of potassium and amino acids, as well as helping to create a more satiating 'meal in a glass'.

Goji berries have all 18 amino acids as well as a good healthy dose of vitamin A (beta carotene), B1, B2, B6and vitamin E. It is believed that Goji berries contain more vitamin C by weight than any other food on Earth!

MAKING A MINT

There are over 30 varieties of mint including Basil Mint, Moroccan Mint, Banana Mint, and even Pineapple Mint.

ORANGE, MINT & SPINACH INFUSION

OK so orange, mint & spinach isn't exactly a combination that immediately springs to mind, but this unlikely combo works well in a juice.

INGREDIENTS:

Orange 1 (peeled, white pith left on)
Cucumber ¼
Spinach Leaves 1 handful
Lime 1 (peeled, white pith left on)
Raw Ginger 3 cm
Fresh Mint 1 small handful
Ice 1 small handful

INSTRUCTIONS:

Simplicity is once again the key, just juice the lot, pour over ice and sip slowly.

JUICING TIP:

If you are using a fast (centrifugal) juicer always remember to tightly pack the spinach and mint in between the harder produce to ensure maximum juice extraction.

However, if you are using a slow (masticating/cold press) juicer then feel free to juice in any order you fancy as these machines are designed to handle leafy greens.

SO WHAT IS IN THIS BABY?

The addition of fresh ginger and fresh mint not only adds that kick you need but also stimulates the senses.

Ginger is made up of many essential nutrients and vitamins, including pyridoxine (vitamin B6) and pantothenic acid (vitamin B5), vitamins that are required for optimum health.

Mint is also a good source of several essential minerals, including magnesium, copper, iron, potassium, and calcium. Magnesium and calcium are both important minerals for bone health.

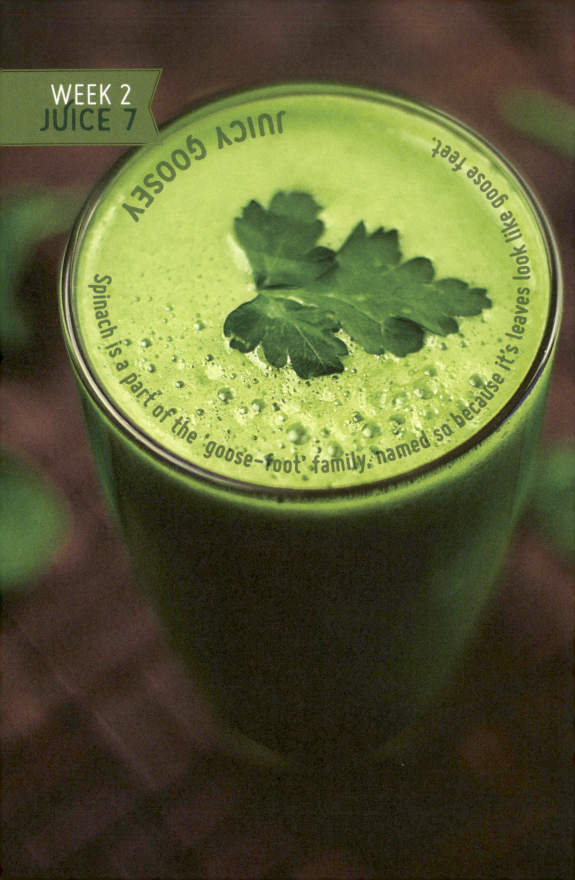

JUICY GOOSEY

Spinach is a part of the 'goose-foot' family, named so because it's leaves look like goose feet.

PARSLEY & LEMON HEALTH HITTER

In cooking, parsley's fragrant leaves are used to enliven and flavour a dish and there is certainly no exception when adding these pungent little leaves to a juice.

INGREDIENTS:

Apple 1
Pear 1
Cucumber 1
Spinach Leaves 1 handful
Lemon ½ (wax free, rind on)
Fresh Parsley 1 small handful
Ice 1 small handful

INSTRUCTIONS:

No need to peel anything, even the lemon rind should be left on for this recipe. All you need to do is juice the lot, pour over ice and enjoy.

JUICING TIP:

If you are using a fast (centrifugal) juicer always remember to tightly pack the spinach and parsley in between the harder produce to ensure maximum juice extraction.

However, if you are using a slow (masticating/cold press) juicer then feel free to juice in any order you fancy as these machines are designed to handle leafy greens.

SO WHAT IS IN THIS BABY?

This juice contains fresh, raw parsley. This earthy little herb, with its bitter notes, really lifts the muted juices of cucumber, pear and apple, whilst leafy green spinach infuses beautifully with a splash of fresh lemon juice.

Parsley is an excellent source of vitamin C, K, E and a good source of vitamin A (notably through its concentration of the provitamin A carotenoid, beta-carotene). It's high in iron and also contains magnesium, potassium and calcium, as well as flavonoids, antioxidants and folic acid.

Spinach is a rich source of vitamin A, the B vitamins riboflavin and vitamin B6, vitamin C, vitamin E and vitamin K.

ODD COMBINATIONS

If you think sweet & sour is an odd combination you could try sprinkling a little black pepper on your strawberries, it's surprisingly tasty.

SWEET + SOUR SENSATION

Forget Chinese 'take-out' and 'take-in' this juicy Sweet & Sour
Sensation instead (minus the guilt and mountains of foil containers!).

INGREDIENTS:

Apples 2
Pear 1
Strawberries 1 small handful
Raw Beetroot 1
Lemon ½ (wax free, rind on)
Lime 1 (peeled, white pith left on)
Ice 1 small handful

INSTRUCTIONS:

Simply juice the beetroot, lemon, lime, apples and pear.

Pour the freshly extracted juice into a blender with
some ice and the strawberries. Whiz until smooth
and voilà!

SO WHAT IS IN THIS BABY?

The earthy sweetness of raw beetroot blends beautifully with luscious red berries, apples and
creamy pear that follow the initial snappy sourness of lemon and lime.

The sweet beetroot in this juice is an excellent source of folate; a B vitamin essential for
numerous bodily functions such as aiding cell growth and producing healthy red blood cells.

The sour lemon is a rich source of vitamin C, one of the most powerful of antioxidants, plus
vitamin B6, riboflavin and thiamine.

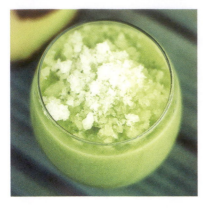
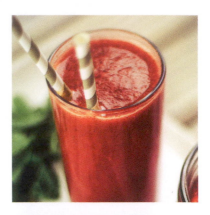
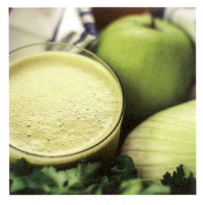
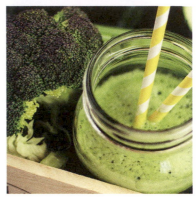

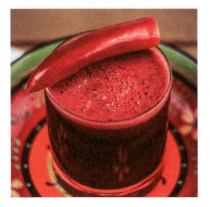
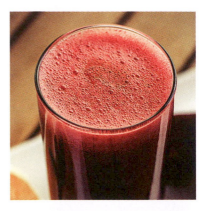
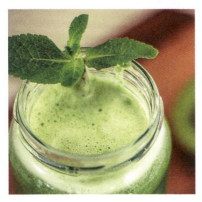
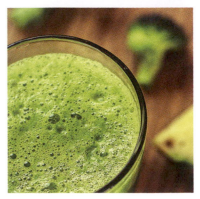

THE JUICES

DAY ONE

FAT LOT OF GOOD

FENNEL EXPRESS

HOT + REDDY

MINTY KIWI REFRESHER

DAY TWO

CARROT, STRAWBERRY, MINT INFUSION

GREEN VEGGIE BIG HITTER

PINK PARADISE

PINEAPPLE, BROCCOLI CRUSH

SHOPPING LIST

Apples (Golden Delicious or Gala)	7	Lemon (unwaxed)	1
Avocado (ripe)	1	Mangetout	6g
Raw Beetroots (small)	2	Orange	1
Broccoli Stem (or use florets)	9cm	Pears	4
Carrots (medium)	2	Pineapple (medium)	1
Celery Stalks	4	Spinach Leaves	45g
Red Chilli	1	Fresh Strawberries	125g
Courgette/Zucchini (medium)	1	Fresh Fennel (small)	½ bulb
Cucumbers (medium)	2	Raw Ginger	30g
Pink Grapefruit	1	Fresh Mint	40g
Kale	24g	Fresh Parsley	10g
Kiwi Fruit	1	Omega 3-6-9 Oil	5ml
Lettuce	¼ head		

GOOD LOT OF FAT

Did you know, the average adult has approximately 50 billion fat cells, which means there are more fat cells in one human body than there are people on planet earth.

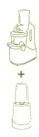

FAT LOT OF GOOD

....and a good lot of fat features in this satiating avocado,
fruit and veggie blend.

INGREDIENTS:

Apples 2
Pear 1
Cucumber ½
Broccoli Stem 3 cm (or use florets)
Lime 1 (peeled, white pith left on)
Avocado ¼ (ripe)
Omega 3-6-9 Oil 1 tsp
Ice 1 small handful

INSTRUCTIONS:

Juice the apples, pear, cucumber, broccoli and lime.

Place the avocado, ice and omega oil into a blender,
pour the juice on top and whiz until beautiful.

Get yourself a lovely glass, sit yourself down
somewhere comfy and enjoy!

SO WHAT IS IN THIS BABY?

Just in case you haven't already read the memo FAT WILL NOT MAKE YOU FAT (well the good,
healthy fats that feature in this programme certainly won't). The unsaturated essential fats
present in this thick and deliciously fulfilling blend are what makes it a pure liquid feast that is
not only heart and joint healthy but super satisfying too.

Omega oils are essential fatty acids (EFA's): the good fats that our body requires. They are
important for maintaining cells, regulating body temperature and healthy immune function.

Mono-unsaturated fats provide nutrients to help develop and maintain the body's cells. Oils rich
in mono-unsaturated fats also contribute vitamin E to the diet, which is a vital antioxidant.
Avocados, olive oil, almonds and macadamia nuts are all a great source of mono-unsaturated
fats.

AN APPLE A DAY

Apparently the average person eats just 65 apples per year... we suspect the average juicer consumes substantially more!

FENNEL EXPRESS

According to Leonardo da Vinci
'Simplicity is the ultimate sophistication'
which is a perfect description for this juice.

INGREDIENTS:

Apple 1
Pear 1
Fennel ½ bulb
Celery 2 stalks
Fresh Parsley 1 small handful
Ice 1 small handful

INSTRUCTIONS:

Simply juice the lot, pour over a little ice and allow your taste buds to get lost in this aniseed sensation.

JUICING TIP:

If you are using a fast (centrifugal) juicer always remember to tightly pack the spinach and mint in between the harder produce to ensure maximum juice extraction.

However, if you are using a slow (masticating/cold press) juicer then feel free to juice in any order you fancy as these machines are designed to handle leafy greens.

SO WHAT IS IN THIS BABY?

Don't let the ease of making this juice distract from the nutritional impact this beauty has once inside the body. The Fennel really lifts an otherwise 'normal' juice and transforms it from black and white to colour.

Fennel is an excellent source of vitamin C and folate; a B vitamin that is said to be essential in helping with the prevention of anaemia. Fennel is also a very rich source of a variety of minerals, including potassium, manganese, copper, phosphorus, calcium, magnesium, niacin and iron.

Although it may look like just a simple piece of fruit, there's actually more to an apple than meets the eye! Apples are full of body boosters including vitamins A, B1, B2, B6, C, E, K, and folate.

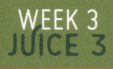

WEIGHT LOSS WONDER
The smell of grapefruit is said to reduce feelings of hunger while the fruit suppresses appetite.

HOT + REDDY

This smoothie really is a unique taste sensation not to be missed.

INGREDIENTS:

Pear 1
Raw Beetroot 1
Pink Grapefruit ¼
(peeled, white pith left on)
Orange 1 (peeled, white pith left on)
Strawberries 1 small handful
Red Chilli ½ (seeds removed!)
Ice 1 small handful

INSTRUCTIONS:

Simply juice this spicy combination and cool off over a little ice. Sip slowly and enjoy.

JUICING TIP:

If you are using a fast (centrifugal) juicer always remember to tightly pack the strawberries in between the harder produce to ensure maximum juice extraction.

However, if you are using a slow (masticating/cold press) juicer then feel free to juice in any order you fancy as these machines are designed to handle berries.

SO WHAT IS IN THIS BABY?

Combining the snap of citrus with the coolness of the beetroot and pear; offset against the sumptuous sweetness of strawberries and hot-headed chilli creates the Hot + Reddy infusion, a true taste sensation!

The humble little raspberry contain a very rich source of vitamin C and dietary fibre; alongside a moderate amount of vitamin K, which is essential in building strong bones. Raspberries also contain a large quantity of manganese, which helps with the absorption of calcium, regulation of blood sugar levels and metabolism.

WHAT'S IN A NAME?

Kiwi Fruit was first called the 'Chinese Gooseberry' until it was changed to reflect where it came from... New Zealand!

MINTY KIWI REFRESHER

Refreshing, light, pure, nutritious and tasty are just a few
of the words I can think of to describe this juice.

INGREDIENTS:

Apples 2
Pear 1
Kiwi Fruit 1 (peeled)
Cucumber ½
Spinach Leaves 1 handful
Fresh Mint 1 small handful
Ice 1 small handful

INSTRUCTIONS:

Juice the ingredients and then pour into a nice glass,
add some ice, and get ready to feel refreshed!

JUICING TIP:

If you are using a fast (centrifugal) juicer always
remember to tightly pack the spinach, kiwi and mint
in between the harder produce to ensure maximum
juice extraction.

However, if you are using a slow (masticating/cold
press) juicer then feel free to juice in any order you
fancy as these machines are designed to handle leafy
greens.

SO WHAT IS IN THIS BABY?

The cucumber, apple and pear juices provide the volume as well soluble fibre, vitamins and
minerals. The mint, spinach and kiwi bring something a little extra to the table.

Spinach is packed full of vitamin K, which is known to be essential for building strong bones,
preventing heart disease and has also been suggested to improve insulin sensitivity. The
abundance of vitamins and minerals found in spinach can also help bring quick relief from dry,
itchy skin and help you maintain a healthy complexion.

Kiwi Fruit is the little fruit holding big surprises, the kiwifruit is a very rich source of vitamin C
as well as vitamin K, vitamin E and provitamin A (beta-carotene).

CARROT CRAZY!

British farmers plant a whopping 22 billion carrot seeds each year, producing 100 carrots per person.

CARROT, STRAWBERRY & MINT INFUSION

I have yet to find a person who doesn't love this recipe. Carrot and Apple juice is one the classics and always goes down well, but the second you add mint and ginger you lift to another level.

INGREDIENTS:

Apple 1
Carrots 2
Strawberries 1 large handful
Raw Ginger 3 cm
Fresh Mint 1 small handful
Ice 1 small handful

INSTRUCTIONS:

Juice the carrots, apple and ginger.

Place the mint leaves and strawberries into a blender with some ice and pour in the juice. Simply blend until smooth, pour and enjoy.

SO WHAT IS IN THIS BABY?

Strawberries are an outstanding source of antioxidant—enhancing vitamin C, as well as vitamin B6 and omega-3 fats. They are also a very good source of iron, copper, potassium, phosphorus and magnesium.

Aromatic and flavoursome raw ginger ticks a great deal of boxes on the health front; including inducing gastrointestinal relief and acting as a great anti-sickness and anti-inflammatory agent.

Fresh mint is a good source of several essential minerals, including magnesium, iron, copper, potassium and calcium.

JE MANGE
Mangetout is a French word meaning 'Eat All' as you eat the young pod with the peas.

GREEN VEGGIE BIG HITTER

I think sometimes we lose touch of the fact that ultimately food
is for fuel and that you are only ever going to get out what
you put in. Put in rubbish and you'll run like a cheap car!
But not on this program and certainly not with this recipe.

INGREDIENTS:

Apple 1
Cucumber ½
Celery 1 stalk
Broccoli Stem 3 cm (or use florets)
Courgette/Zucchini ½
Mangetout 6
Spinach Leaves 1 handful
Kale 1 handful
Lettuce 1 small handful
Ice 1 small handful

INSTRUCTIONS:

Simply juice the lot and pour over a little ice, then
turn your phone and laptop off and take 5 minutes
for yourself.

JUICING TIP:

If you are using a fast (centrifugal) juicer always
remember to tightly pack the leafy greens in
between the harder produce to ensure maximum
juice extraction.

However, if you are using a slow (masticating/cold
press) juicer then feel free to juice in any order you
fancy as these machines are designed to handle leafy
greens.

SO WHAT IS IN THIS BABY?

Consuming the freshly extracted juices from natures finest fruits, but even more so, vegetables,
will have you running like a Ferrari! Mineral rich leafy greens; the bitter twist of mangetout,
gently sweetened with apple, cucumber and courgette. This is the nutritional hit that will keep
on giving.

Depending on the variety, lettuce is a very good source of vitamin A, vitamin K and folate, with
higher concentrations of vitamin A found in darker lettuce leaves. Lettuce also provides calcium,
iron, copper and manganese, with vitamins and minerals largely found in the leaf.

Sweet and juicy mangetout is a member of the pea family and is rich in vitamin A and vitamin C,
as well as vitamin K and folate.

PINEAPPLE PLANTS
You can actually grow your own pineapple plant from the top of your pineapple, however it takes 2-3 years to produce fruit so you might want to stick to buying them.

PINK PARADISE

Pineapple and grapefruit has been the perfect combination of a certain famous 'fizzy and sugary' canned drink for years. That's because these two fruits compliment each other beautifully.

INGREDIENTS:

Pink Grapefruit ½
(peeled, white pith left on)
Pineapple ½ (peeled)
Raw Beetroot 1
Fresh Mint 1 small handful
Ice 1 small handful

INSTRUCTIONS:

Simply juice everything and pour over ice.

JUICING TIP:

If you are using a fast (centrifugal) juicer always remember to tightly pack the mint in between the harder produce to ensure maximum juice extraction.

However, if you are using a slow (masticating/cold press) juicer then feel free to juice in any order you fancy as these machines are designed to handle leafy greens.

SO WHAT IS IN THIS BABY?

I wanted to make a juice which had the spirit of a certain famous drink but without the sugar and chemicals. I also wanted to add some additional ingredients to lift it on the health front and freshly extracted beetroot and mint juice fitted that bill perfectly.

Renowned for their tart and tangy taste, the juicy pink grapefruit provides an excellent source of vitamin C, vitamin A and vitamin B1. It is also a good source of pantothenic acid, copper, potassium and biotin, which has been said to help maintain a steady blood sugar level.

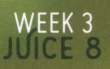

POTENT CELERY

It takes just one ounce of celery seeds to produce an acre of celery.

PINEAPPLE, BROCCOLI CRUSH

There are few juices on earth that match either the texture or taste
of freshly extracted pineapple juice. It adds a deliciously creamy top
and a sweetness that no other fruit or vegetable can match.

INGREDIENTS:

Celery 1 stalk
Cucumber ½
Broccoli Stem 3 cm (or use florets)
Pineapple ½ (peeled)
Ice 1 small handful

INSTRUCTIONS:

Simply juice the lot, pour over the crushed ice and
enjoy!

SO WHAT IS IN THIS BABY?

I've added the 'super food' broccoli for maximum nutrition; cucumber for it's natural diuretic
ability and celery for sodium. For those who claim 'it can't be good for you if it tastes good'
needs to try this baby on for size!

The brilliant broccoli is high in vitamin C, vitamin K, which is required in the body for healthy
blood coagulation, folate, riboflavin , vitamin B6 and thiamine. It's a very good source of minerals
such as potassium, copper, magnesium, zinc, calcium and iron.

Celery contains a good source of vitamin B2, vitamin C, vitamin B6, and vitamin A in the form of
carotenoids, which are said to be beneficial for decreasing the risk of disease.

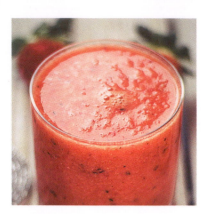
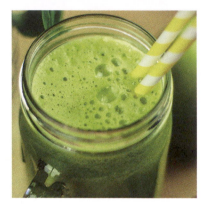
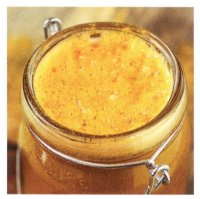
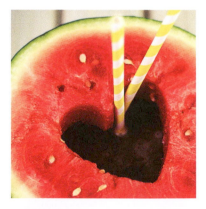
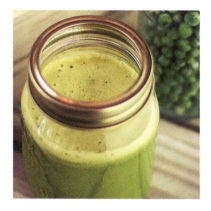
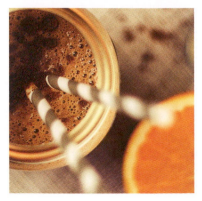
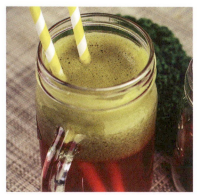
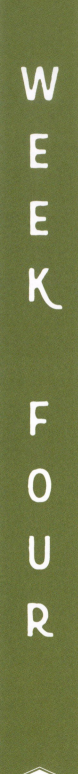

WEEK FOUR

THE JUICES

DAY ONE

9am   CARIBBEAN POWER BLEND

1pm   TURMERIC TEMPTATION

4pm   EASY PEASY LEMON SQUEEZY

7pm   KALE, RASPBERRY,
STRAWBERRY AID

DAY TWO

9am   LOVE JUICE

1pm   HERBIPHWOARRRR!

4pm   WATERMELON, MINT COOLER

7pm   CHOCOLATE ORANGE
POWER BLEND

SHOPPING LIST

Apples (Golden Delicious or Gala)	5	Fresh Garden Peas	90g
Banana (ripe and Fair-Trade)	1	Pineapple (medium)	1
Carrots (medium)	2	Fresh Raspberries	60g
Celery Stalks	2	Fresh Strawberries	60g
Cucumbers (medium)	2	Watermelon (medium)	1
Kale	24g	Fresh Basil	40g
Lemon (unwaxed)	2	Fresh Mint	125g
Limes (unwaxed)	1	Fresh Parsley	10g
Mango (ripe)	1	Raw Turmeric (or powdered)	30g
Oranges (large)	4	Cocoa Powder	2.5g
Papaya	1	Maca Powder	2.5g
Passion Fruits	2	Coconut Water	350ml
Pears	4	Manuka Honey	10g

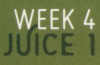

SPICY PEPPAYA

Papaya seeds are edible and have a spicy peppery taste that can be used as a substitute for black pepper.

CARIBBEAN POWER BLEND

Imagine lying on deserted beach, turquoise seas reaching out as far as the eye can see. You feel the powdery white sand beneath you as the waves lap at your feet and the cool sea breeze brushes your face... bliss!

INGREDIENTS:

Mango 60 g (peeled & diced)
Papaya 60 g (peeled & diced)
Pineapple 60 g (peeled & diced)
Coconut Water 350 ml
Lime 1
Ice 1 small handful

INSTRUCTIONS:

If it seems a little odd that we have started instructing with weight rather than our usual juicy measurements, it's purely because the size of Mangos and Papayas vary so much. To make sure you made the correct amount of juice we thought we would be fancy and dig our scales out.

Place all ingredients (apart from the lime) into the blender.

Cut the lime in half and squeeze the juice from both halves into the blender. Then all you need to do is blend until smooth, pour and enjoy!

SO WHAT IS IN THIS BABY?

Ripe and fleshy mango, refreshing coconut water, the tropical taste sensations of pineapple and papaya and a squeeze of fresh lime, your own little bit of paradise in a glass!

MANGO & PAPAYA TIP:

To easily remove the large flat 'stone' place the mango on its side and cut it slightly off centre so you miss the stone as you cut through. Take the mango half and 'score' into cubes, turn the mango inside out and cut the pieces from the skin. Repeat on the other side.

Papayas do not have a stone but they do have a lot of seeds so make sure you remove before scooping out the papaya flesh.

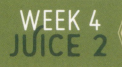

TURMERIC TEA

Okinawa in Japan has the world's longest life span which some attribute to their habit of daily drinking turmeric tea.

TURMERIC TEMPTATION

You won't be surprised to hear that turmeric comes from the same family as ginger, especially after tasting this.

INGREDIENTS:

Apple 1
Pear 1
Carrots 2
Cucumber ½
Raw Turmeric 3 cm
(or a generous pinch of powder)
Ice 1 small handful

INSTRUCTIONS:

No need to peel a thing, simply juice the lot, pour into a lovely glass over ice. Grab a good book, find somewhere comfy to sit and drink slowly.

JUICING TIP:

If using powdered turmeric, simply add a pinch to the freshly extracted juice and stir in. Alternatively you could give it a shake in a shaker bottle or a whiz in the blender.

SO WHAT IS IN THIS BABY?

Like ginger, turmeric adds an aromatic warmth but with a slight peppery undertone. Less is definitely more with this pungent little spice, which uplifts the subtle flavours of juicy apple, pear, cool cucumber and crisp carrots.

JUICY INGREDIENT NOTE:

At time of writing this book, getting hold of raw turmeric root isn't easy. Having said that, if you live in say London or New York (or a similar hub of the new and cool), many trendy health food shops keep a stock and you can also find it online at reputable stores. However if you can't get hold of any then simply replace fresh and raw with a good quality turmeric powder.

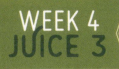

PEAS BE PEA-LITE

The correct way to eat your peas is to squash them on the back of your fork... but we don't expect you to put them in your juicer like that!

EASY, PEASY LEMON SQUEEZY

All we ask is that you give peas a chance (see what we did there!).
Seriously this juice, with its simple garden variety ingredients,
tastes out of the park.

INGREDIENTS:

Apple 1
Pear 1
Cucumber ¼
Fresh Garden Peas 1 large handful
Lemon ½ (wax free, rind on)
Ice 1 small handful

INSTRUCTIONS:

True to its name it couldn't be easier — just juice the lot, no need to peel anything! Pour into a nice glass, kick off your shoes, pull up a chair and take your time over this surprisingly tasty juice.

JUICING TIP:

If you are using a fast (centrifugal) juicer always remember to tightly pack the peas in between the harder produce to ensure maximum juice extraction.

However, if you are using a slow (masticating/cold press) juicer then feel free to juice in any order you fancy as these machines are designed to handle peas.

SO WHAT IS IN THIS BABY?

Fresh, fruity and full of flavour, this pure and simple concoction will benefit your skin, hair, nails and help to give you an all over body cleanse, inside and out.

Little green peas pack a great punch in terms of nutrients, and are a very good source of vitamin K, vitamin B1, vitamin B6 and folate. While not always recognised as a food unique in phytonutrients, green peas are actually a fantastic source,including flavanols, phenolic acid and carotenoids. They are also a great source of copper, iron, potassium and magnesium.

Cucumbers are an excellent source of vitamin K, vitamin C and vitamin B1 (also known as thiamine), which has been said to help boost the immune system and aid digestive problems.

50 SHADE OF KALE

There are many varieties of kale,

Curly Kale, Red Russian Kale

and even Dinosaur Kale.

KALE, RASPBERRY & STRAWBERRY AID

Yes you did read correctly, I have combined berries with kale!

INGREDIENTS:

Apples 2
Kale 1 handful
Raspberries 1 small handful
Strawberries 1 small handful
Cucumber ¼
Lemon ⅓ (wax free, rind on)
Ice 1 small handful

INSTRUCTIONS:

Simply juice the lot and pour over ice. Stir regularly as you drink to combine the juice as this one has a tendency to separate (as you can see from the picture).

JUICING TIP:

If you are using a fast (centrifugal) juicer always remember to tightly pack the kale, raspberries and strawberries in between the harder produce to ensure maximum juice extraction.

However, if you are using a slow (masticating/cold press) juicer then feel free to juice in any order you fancy as these machines are designed to handle leafy greens and berries.

SO WHAT IS IN THIS BABY?

The thing I love most about juicing is the amount of nutrition you can 'hide'. Which means you can still absorb all the goodness without having to compromise on taste. This recipe really is no exception. Kale is loaded with all the 'good stuff' our bodies are crying out for, but is disguised perfectly amongst the sweet crunch of apples, succulent berries, the subtle purity of fresh cucumber juice and lively lemon. Try it on your kids, after all what they know won't hurt them!

JUICY INGREDIENT NOTE:

If you can't get hold of kale you can use spinach, cabbage or other dark leafy greens.

PASSIONATE FRUIT

Passion fruit are green when young, changing to shades of red purple or yellow as they ripen.

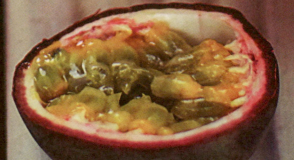

LOVE JUICE

This glass of romance will certainly tickle your taste buds. Plump red berries intimately blended with the gentle tropical crunch of passion fruit and creamy fresh orange juice, guaranteed to satiate and satisfy your appetite.

INGREDIENTS:

Strawberries 1 small handful
Raspberries 1 small handful
Passion Fruits 2
Oranges 2 (peeled, white pith left on)
Ice 1 small handful

INSTRUCTIONS:

Juice the oranges and pour into blender.

Cut the passion fruits in half and spoon out the insides, including the seeds, and place into a blender.

Add the berries and some ice.

Whiz until smooth, pour into a glass and feel the love.

SO WHAT IS IN THIS BABY?

This smoothie will take your breath away with the first taste. Juicy passion fruit is a fabulous source of vitamin A, vitamin E, vitamin C and B vitamins including riboflavin. Passion fruit contains excellent sources of iron, phosphorus, potassium and magnesium, as well as calcium and zinc.

Strawberries are an excellent source of antioxidant-promoting vitamin C, which helps to protect cells, maintain healthy connective tissue within the body and can also help with wound healing. Strawberries also contain an excellent source of the mineral manganese, which is said to promote a healthy bone structure by helping to create essential enzymes for building bones.

BRILLIANT BASIL

There are many of varieties of Basil, the most common being 'Sweet Basil' which is the one sold in most grocery stores.

HERBIPHWOARRRR!

Two incredibly nutritious and powerful herbs (or errrbs if in the US!)
feature in this surprisingly delicious green juice.

INGREDIENTS:

Apple 1
Pear 1
Celery 2 stalks
Cucumber ¼
Lemon ½ (wax free, rind on)
Fresh Basil 1 large handful
Fresh Parsley 1 small handful
Ice 1 small handful

INSTRUCTIONS:

Couldn't be easier. Juice the lot, pour into a lovely glass
over ice, grab a bean bag and sit ye down. Oh and of
course enjoy!

JUICING TIP:

If you are using a fast (centrifugal) juicer always
remember to tightly pack the leafy greens in
between the harder produce to ensure maximum
juice extraction.

However, if you are using a slow (masticating/cold
press) juicer then feel free to juice in any order you
fancy as these machines are designed to handle leafy
greens.

SO WHAT IS IN THIS BABY?

Parsley juice is particularly potent, so you need very little of this herb to pack a punch. However,
you can be generous with the basil and it's this gorgeous herb that adds the 'Phwoarrr' to this
rather cornily named 'Herbiphwoarrrr!' juice. The apple, pear and cucumber are all there to
add natural sweetness, as well as insoluble fibre and the lemon just balances the whole juice
beautifully.

Fresh basil is an excellent source of vitamin A (in the form of carotenoids, such as beta-
carotene), vitamin C and vitamin K. Basil is a great source of calcium, iron, folate, magnesium,
manganese and copper.

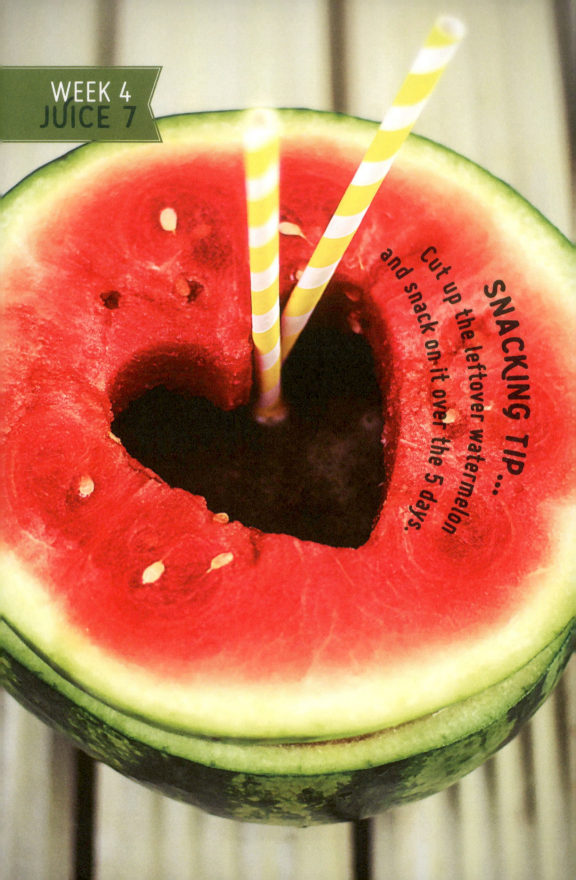

SNACKING TIP...
Cut up the leftover watermelon and snack on it over the 5 days.

WATERMELON, MINT COOLER

The old adage of 'don't judge a book by its cover' is perfectly apt here.

INGREDIENTS:

Pear 1
Cucumber ½
Watermelon ⅛ (keep the skin on)
Fresh Mint 1 small handful
Ice 1 small handful

INSTRUCTIONS:

Juice all the ingredients and pour over ice — simple!

JUICING TIP:

Watermelons come in all sizes. I have given an amount of one eighth of a small watermelon for this recipe, but feel free to not get too caught up on it. Think of a nice 6cm slice of watermelon and you'll have the size I am trying to describe.

SO WHAT IS IN THIS BABY?

Watermelon, when juiced with the skin on, turns the whole juice a slightly muddy colour. However, do not let this put you off, as the colour doesn't match the taste. This is bursting with flavour, incredibly cooling to the system, it's rich in zinc, SO good for the skin and is just a little bit different. It's also full of vitamin C, vitamin A in the form of carotenoids and vitamins B1 and B6.

The combination of watermelon and cucumber makes this juice ridiculously hydrating and I can't stress the importance of ensuring you remain well hydrated. The body is unable to distinguish between hunger and thirst; a lot of the time we think we're hungry when we're actually just thirsty!

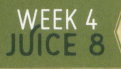
CHOCCATASTIC!

Cocoa Beans are the seeds found inside the pods of the Cacao tree, each pod contains enough beans for 2 bars of dark chocolate.

CHOCOLATE, ORANGE POWER BLEND

Chocolate orange doesn't have to be exclusively for cakes
of the Jaffa variety or set within over-processed
milk chocolate and wrapped in orange foil.

INGREDIENTS:

Oranges 2 (peeled, white pith left on)
Banana 1 (ripe)
Cocoa Powder 1 heaped tsp
Maca Powder ½ tsp
Manuka Honey 1 tsp
Ice 1 small handful

INSTRUCTIONS:

Juice the oranges and pour into a blender.

Put the banana, cocoa powder, maca powder, manuka honey and ice into the blender.

Blend until smooth, drink and enjoy this ridiculously tasty smoothie!

SO WHAT IS IN THIS BABY?

This chocolatey glass of goodness tastes like a naughty treat and is actually good for you! The sweetness of manuka honey offsets the bitterness of cocoa whilst the butterscotch tones of maca really boost, not only the flavour, but more importantly the nutrition, powering this blend with even more vitamins, minerals, enzymes and essential amino acids.

Cocoa powder contains several minerals including copper, magnesium, phosphorus, potassium, sodium and zinc; as well iron and calcium.

Maca, a root that belongs to the radish family, is most commonly ground into a powder that is rich in vitamin C, vitamin B and vitamin E. Maca powder provides plenty of calcium, zinc, magnesium and iron, which helps restore red blood cells.

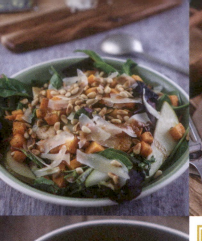
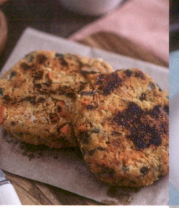
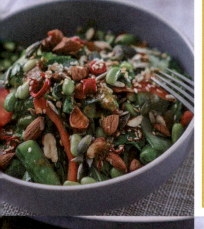
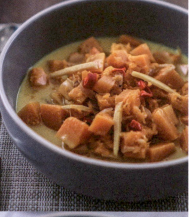
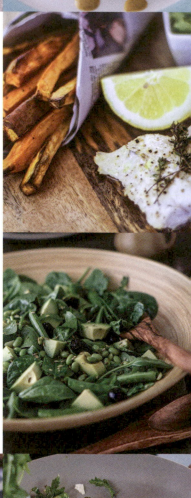

SALADS

VEGAN

VEGETARIAN

FISH

SUPER FAST FOOD

FOR THE DAYS WHEN YOU WANT TO USE YOUR TEETH!

The following recipes are all taken from my first ever cookbook 'SUPER fast FOOD'. I have included them in this book in order to give you an idea of the sort of 'clean' meals you can incorporate into the days when you're using your teeth.

These recipes are all examples of what I describe as 'Low H. I. Food' (Human Intervention) In other words, the less a human interferes with your food, the healthier and 'cleaner' it tends to be. Low H. I eating should make up the vast majority of your diet and if you juice for two days a week, eat clean for three and then be 'human' for two, you'll be guaranteeing the vast majority of what's going into your body will indeed be Low H. I.

Yes there are Super Food Salads, as you'd expect, but there's also my version of Fish 'n' Chips and, in the main hardback book, there's even a Super Food veggie burger. This all goes to show that eating 'clean' doesn't have to equal boring and unadventurous.

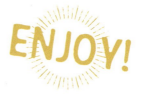

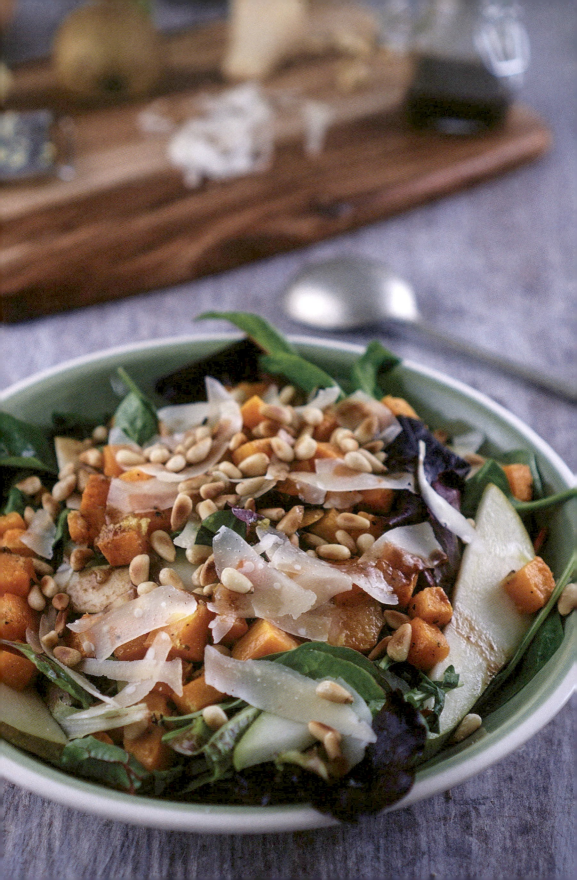

WARM GINGER INFUSED BUTTERNUT SQUASH WITH PEAR, PARMESAN & TOASTED PINE NUTS. SERVED WITH AN ORANGE, HONEY & BALSAMIC REDUCTION.

This truly gorgeous salad works equally as well in winter as it does in summer. Light, sweet and packing a little heat, it genuinely has it all. Butternut squash, with its mild nutty flavour is super satiating and loaded with vitamin A, largely in the form of beta-carotene, fibre, potassium and magnesium. It may take a little longer to make than the other salads on the menu, but to coin a phrase from a very well known Irish stout 'sometimes good things come to those who wait!'

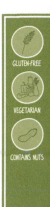

SALAD INGREDIENTS

Serves 2

Butternut Squash ½ small
Olive Oil 2 tablespoon or 30ml
Himalayan Rock Salt 1 pinch
Ground Black Pepper 1 generous pinch
Ginger 4cm x 4cm chunk or 40g
Pear 1
Parmesan or Parmigiano Reggiano Cheese 75g
Mixed Leaves 2 handfuls or 75g
Pine Nuts 1 handful or 50g

REDUCTION INGREDIENTS

Oranges 2
Balsamic Vinegar 4 tablespoons or 60ml

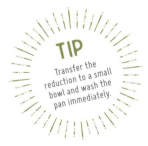

TIP
Transfer the reduction to a small bowl and wash the pan immediately.

PREPARE THE REDUCTION

Juice the oranges directly into a small saucepan and add the vinegar. Gently simmer over a medium to low heat with the lid off for 30 minutes, until the mixture has reduced and slightly thickened.

PREPARE THE SALAD

Preheat the oven to 180°C / gas mark 4. Remove the ends from the butternut squash and peel. Cut in half, remove the seeds and chop into bite sized chunks (about 1cm x 1cm), then scatter onto a baking tray. Drizzle over half the oil and sprinkle over the salt and pepper. Peel, then grate the ginger directly onto the butternut squash and mix so that the squash is coated in oil and seasoning.

COOK

Place the tray in the oven for 30-35 minutes until the squash is cooked.

PREPARE

Cut the pear into quarters, remove the core and slice into thin strips. Shave the cheese with a vegetable peeler into very thin slivers.Put the mixed leaves into a salad bowl; add the pear, remaining olive oil and lightly toss.

WARM

When the butternut squash is cooked, remove from the over. Heat a dry frying pan on the hob and toast the pine nuts for 2-3 minutes over a medium heat until golden, stirring continually, to avoid burning!

SERVE

Put the salad leaves and pear onto a plate, add the butternut squash, cheese and pine nuts. Finish with a generous drizzle of the balsamic reduction.

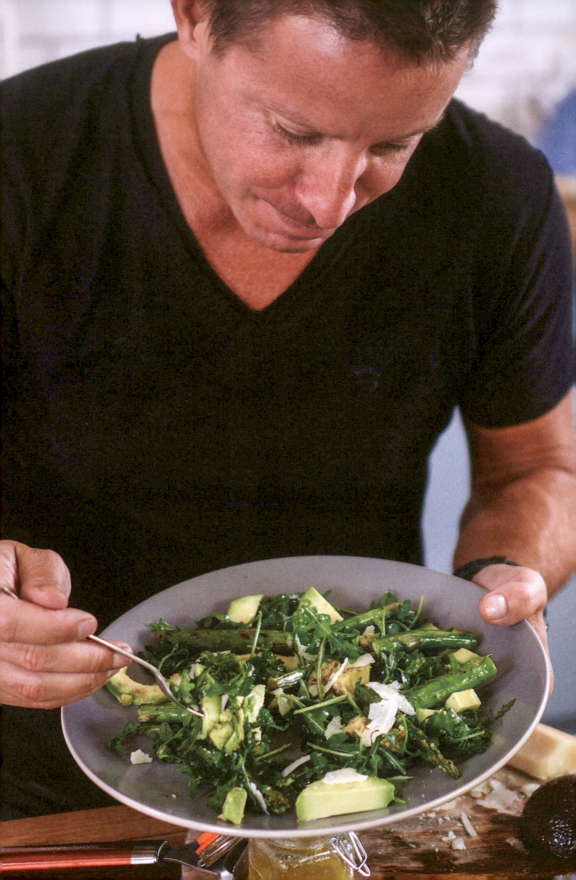

ROCKET, AVOCADO, GRILLED ASPARAGUS & SHAVED PARMESAN WITH A ROASTED GARLIC, LEMON & HONEY DRESSING

A seemingly simple combination of ingredients, but don't let that fool you as this baby delivers nutritionally and tastes sublime. Light, filling and fresh it packs in an unbelievable array of essential nutrients including vitamins, minerals, amino acids, enzymes, good carbohydrates and healthy fats. It's fusion of flavours and tantalizing textures knocks this recipe out the park!

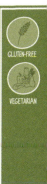

GLUTEN-FREE

VEGETARIAN

INGREDIENTS

Serves 2

Asparagus 8 spears or 140g
Olive Oil 2 tablespoons or 30ml
Ground Black Pepper
1 generous pinch
Avocado 2 medium (ripe)
Parmesan or Parmigiano Reggiano
Cheese 75g
Rocket 2 large handfuls or 100g

DRESSING INGREDIENTS

Garlic 2 cloves (skin on)
Lemon ½
Olive Oil 3 tablespoons or 45ml
Honey 1 teaspoon or 5ml

PREPARE THE DRESSING

Preheat the oven to 180°C / gas mark 4.

Place the cloves of garlic onto a baking tray with the skin on and cook for 5 minutes.

CREATE THE DRESSING

Remove the garlic from the oven, carefully peel (it's hot!) and remove any hard ends. Add to the small mixing container of a hand blender (making sure the blade is already in). Squeeze the lemon juice directly into the container, then add the oil and honey. Blitz for 20 seconds.

CREATE THE SALAD

Remove any hard ends from the asparagus, cut in half and place on a plate. Pour over half the olive oil, sprinkle with the black pepper, turning each piece so it is coated in the olive oil. Cut the avocados in half; remove the stones, scoop out the flesh and cut into generous slices. Shave the cheese with a vegetable peeler into very thin slices. Put the rocket into a bowl, drizzle over the remaining olive oil and lightly toss.

COOK

Heat a griddle pan on a hot ring, add the asparagus and allow to cook for 2-3 minutes before turning and cooking for a further 2-3 minutes.

SERVE

Place the rocket onto the middle of a plate, add the avocado, asparagus and cheese and drizzle over the dressing.

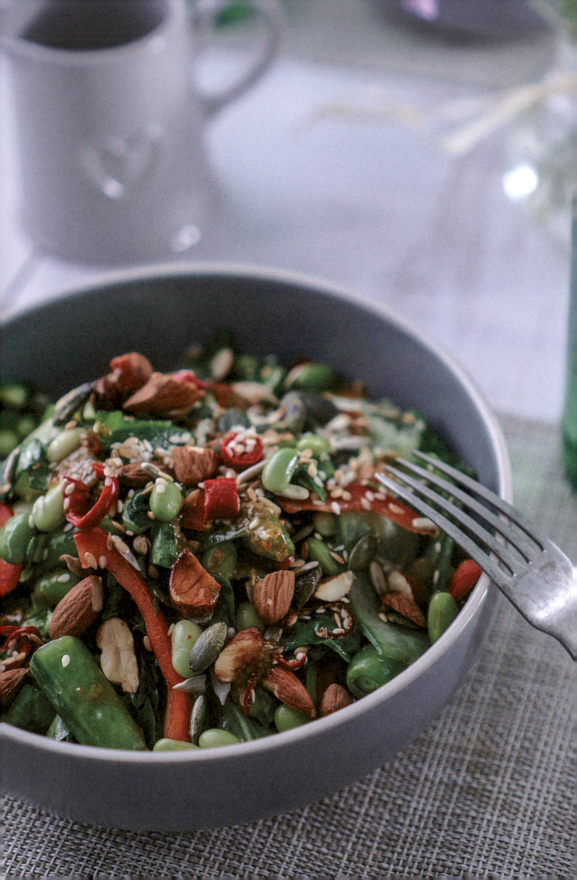

CRUNCHY MUNCHIE SALAD WITH A LIME, CHILLI & CORIANDER DRESSING

As the name suggests, this is one salad you can really get your teeth into and your body will be thankful you did. Loaded with vitamins A, B, C, E, and K as well as magnesium, iron, calcium and manganese this snappy salad is also brimming with phytonutrients proven to have anti-inflammatory properties. Like all the recipes in this book — no chef required and hopefully after a few more meals like this one, no doctor required either!

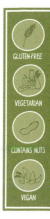

INGREDIENTS

Serves 2

Red Pepper 1 medium
Cucumber ¼ medium
Baby Leaf Spinach 1 large handful or 60g
Sugar Snap Peas 1 handful or 40g
Fresh Edamame Beans 100g
Red Chilli 1 medium
Almonds (whole) 1 handful or 50g
Mixed Seeds 1 large handful or 100g
Himalayan Rock Salt 1 generous pinch

DRESSING INGREDIENTS

Red Chilli 1 medium
Coriander 1 small handful or 20g
Apple Cider Vinegar 1 tablespoon or 15ml
Olive Oil 3 tablespoons or 45ml
Lime ½

CREATE THE DRESSING

Remove the top from the chilli, slice in half lengthways, remove the seeds and place in the mixing container of a hand blender (making sure the blade is already in). Add the other ingredients, squeezing the lime juice directly into the container. Blitz for 10-20 seconds

PREPARE THE SALAD

Preheat the oven to 180°C / gas mark 4.

Finely slice the red pepper, removing the seeds and core. Using a vegetable peeler, slice the cucumber lengthways to create very thin strips (discarding any slices that are just skin). Chop the spinach. Remove the ends from the sugar snap peas and any stringy bits from the spine, then cut in half. Remove the top from the chilli, cut in half, remove the seeds, and slice finely. Coarsely chop the almonds and place on a backing tray along with the chilli, mixed seeds and the salt.

HEAT

Place the baking tray in the oven and cook for 5 minutes

COMBINE

Put all the ingredients; along with the dressing into a salad bowl and mix thoroughly.

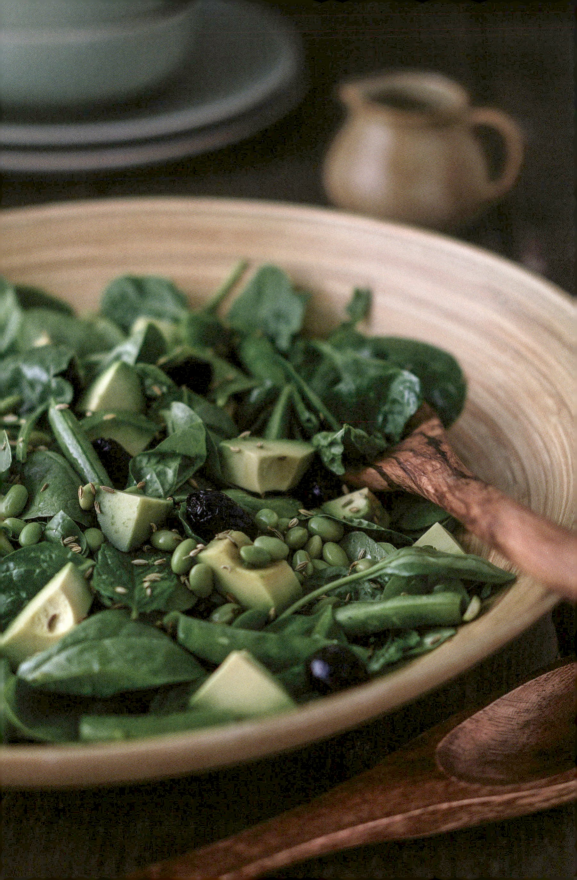

AVOCADO, MINT, FENNEL & EDAMAME SALAD WITH A GINGER, HONEY & YOGHURT SPLASH.

For me, avocado is the world's number one 'super food'. It's so rich, so creamy and yet mind-blowingly nutritious that it should be a staple in everyone's diet. In fact the avocado alone brings to the table in excess of 25 essential nutrients including vitamins A, B, C, E, K, copper, iron, phosphorous magnesium and potassium. The addition of fresh mint, fennel, ginger and honey takes this already delicious dish to a fragrant new level where your taste buds and body will forever wish to remain!

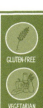

GLUTEN-FREE

VEGETARIAN

INGREDIENTS

Serves 2

Avocado 1 large (ripe)
Sugar Snap Peas or Mange Tout
1 handful or 60g
Fresh Mint 1 small handful
or 20g
Baby Leaf Spinach 2 large
handfuls or 100g
Olive Oil 1 tablespoon or 15ml
Fennel Seeds 1 tablespoon
or 5g
Olives 1 large handful
70g (pitted)
Edamame Beans 1 handful
or 50g

SPLASH INGREDIENTS

Ginger 1cm x 2cm or 10g
Natural Yogurt 3 tablespoons
or 45g
Honey 1 teaspoon or 5ml

CREATE THE DRESSING

Peel the ginger, chop into several pieces and place in the small mixing container of a hand blender (ensure the blade is already in). Add the yoghurt and honey and pulse for 20 seconds.

PREPARE THE SALAD

Cut the avocado in half, remove the stone, scoop out the flesh and cut into nice large chunks. Remove the ends and the stringy spine from the sugar snap peas. Remove the leaves from the mint and discard the stalks.

COMBINE

Put the mint, spinach and sugar snap peas into a bowl, along with the olive oil and fennel seeds and mix. Place the salad onto the plates and add the avocado, olives and edamame beans, then drizzle with the dressing.

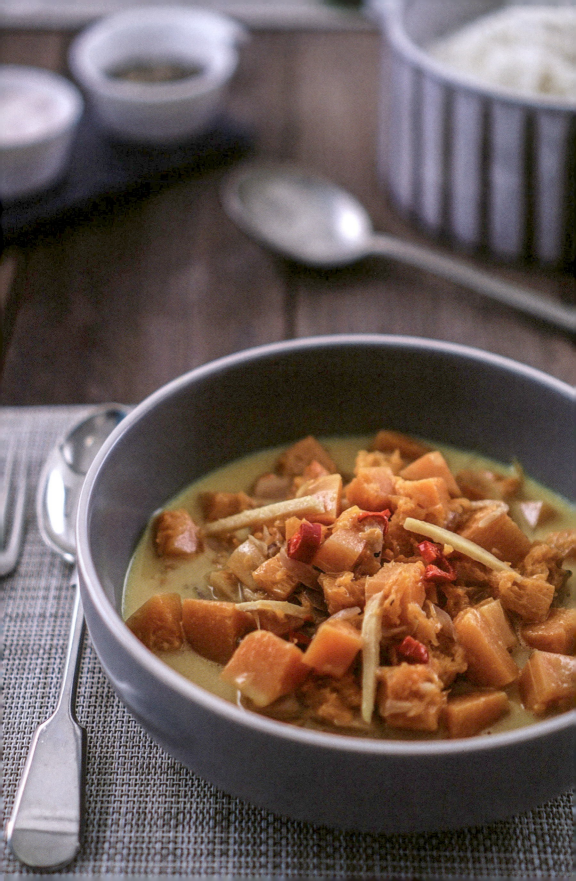

BUTTERNUT SQUASH, CHILLI, GINGER, LIME & COCONUT CURRY ON A BED OF CAULIFLOWER 'RICE'*

Don't knock it till you've tried it is the message here. Personally, I am not the biggest cauliflower fan, yet make it into 'rice' alongside a beautiful spicy butternut squash curry and boom! DELICIOUS! Cauliflower is rich in anti-inflammatory nutrients including vitamin K, and has been studied a great deal in the prevention of cancer. Overall, I would day this is one of the tastiest and 'super food' rich recipes in the whole book.

GLUTEN-FREE

VEGETARIAN

VEGAN

INGREDIENTS

Serves 2

Butternut Squash ½ medium
Red Onion ½ medium
Garlic 2 cloves
Red Chilli 1 medium
Ginger 2cm x 4cm piece or 30g
Lime 1
Coconut Oil 1 tablespoon or 15ml
Coconut Milk 1 tin (400ml)
Turmeric ½ teaspoon

CAULIFLOWER 'RICE' INGREDIENTS

Cauliflower 1 large
Olive Oil 1 tablespoon or 15ml
Himalayan Rock Salt 1 pinch
Ground Black Pepper
1 generous pinch

PREPARE THE CURRY

Remove the end and peel the butternut squash, then remove the seeds and then cut into bite sized chunks. Remove the ends and skin from the red onion and garlic and thinly slice. Remove the top from the chilli, cut in half, remove the seeds and then cut into thin slices. Peel the ginger and cut into matchstick strips. Cut the lime in half.

COOK

Put the coconut oil in a wok or large frying pan and place over a medium heat. Add the butternut squash and cook for 10 minutes stirring occasionally. Then add the onion, chilli and garlic and cook for a further 10 minutes. Next add the coconut milk, turmeric and squeeze the lime directly into the pan. Reduce the heat and allow to simmer for 10 minutes.

MAKE THE CAULIFLOWER RICE

Remove the green leaves from the cauliflower and cut into quarters. Place in a food processor and pulse until all the cauliflower is broken down and resembles cooked rice. If you don't have a food processor you can do this in small batches using a hand blender, the Super Blend or a bullet style blender. You could also grate the cauliflower using the large holes of a traditional grater.

HEAT

Put the olive oil in the pan over a medium heat and then add the cauliflower, salt and pepper and cook for 5 minutes, stirring frequently.

SERVE

Scoop a generous spoonful or two of the 'rice' and curry into a bowl.

*You can obviously use regular rice and simply cook this according to the packet instructions if you prefer.

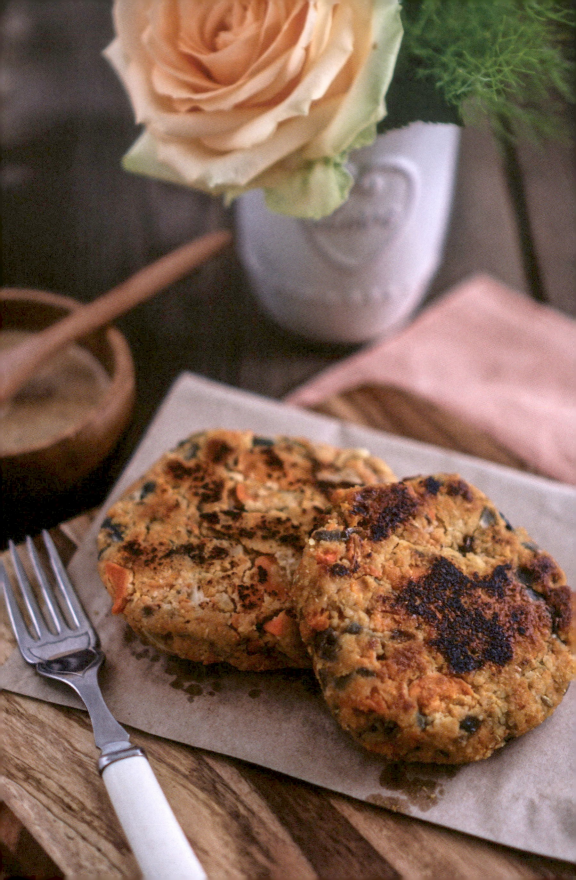

SWEET POTATO CAKES WITH AN ALMOND & LEMON DRIZZLE

If you have recently ventured down the vegan path and used to love fishcakes, then this vegan friendly recipe is the perfect alternative. They work well as a dish in themselves, or why not add a cheeky side order of sweet potato wedges to raise the game. This simple recipe will feed you from the inside out with its generous quantities of vitamins A, B6, C, E and minerals including calcium, iron and magnesium..

POTATO CAKE INGREDIENTS

Serves 2

Sweet Potato 2 medium
Carrot 1 medium
Red Onion ½ medium
Garlic 2 cloves
Almonds 2 handfuls or 100g
Fennel Seeds 1 tablespoon
Olive Oil 1 tablespoon or 15ml
Ground Black Pepper
1 generous pinch
Himalayan Rock Salt 1 pinch

DRIZZLE INGREDIENTS

Lemon ¼
Water 1 tablespoon (15ml)
Almond Butter 2 teaspoons

POTATO CAKE PREP

Preheat the oven to 180°C / gas mark 4.

Remove any hard ends from the potatoes, carrot, onion and garlic, then peel and chop into small chunks. Using either a food processor or hand blender with container attachment, blitz the almonds and fennel seeds for 10–20 seconds until they turn into 'flour'.

COOK

Place the sweet potato, carrot, onion and garlic onto a baking tray, drizzle with the olive oil and mix so all the veg are coated. Place in the oven for 30 minutes stirring part way through.

MAKE THE DRIZZLE

Squeeze the juice of the lemon into a small bowl; add the water and almond butter and combine

CREATE THE POTATO CAKES

Put the cooked vegetables, almond 'flour', salt and pepper into a pan (set the baking tray to one side, but do not wash and do not turn the oven off) and mash using a potato masher. Then divide the mixture and shape into 4 'burgers' and place on the baking tray and pop back in the oven.

COOK

Cook for 15 minutes.

SERVE

Place the potato cakes on a plate and drizzle with the dressing.

GLUTEN-FREE

VEGETARIAN

VEGAN

CONTAINS NUTS

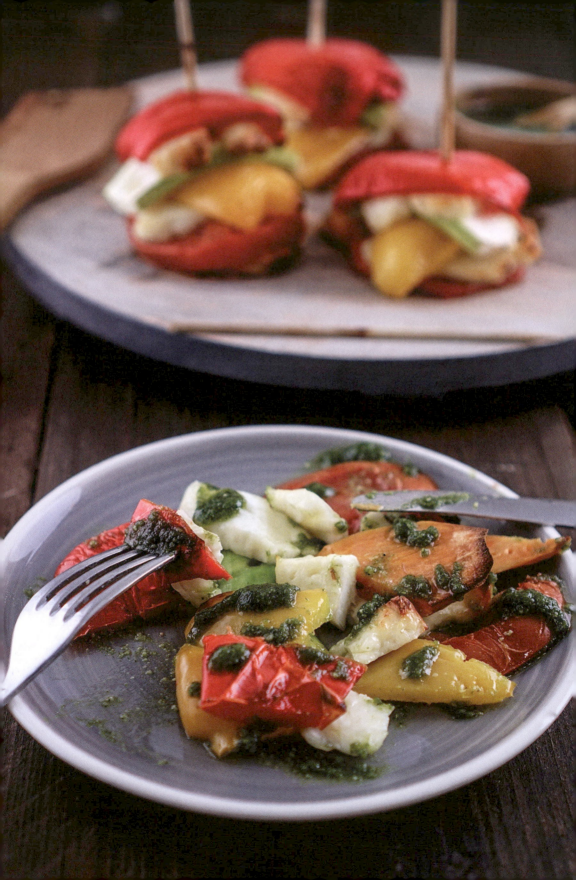

GRILLED HALLOUMI & VEGETABLE STACK, DRIZZLED WITH A LEMON PESTO DRESSING

This recipe taps into those taste buds and is one of my favourites in the book. It's also one I revisit time and time again and I have a feeling you will too. I was a vegan for over four years and the one thing I missed the most was cheese, none more so than warm halloumi. Not only does it add the edge on flavour but is also an excellent source of protein and calcium. Juicy beef tomato and vibrant peppers sweeten this dish up a treat and ramp up those much-needed vitamins A and C.

GLUTEN-FREE

VEGETARIAN

CONTAINS NUTS

INGREDIENTS FOR THE STACKS

Serves 2

Courgette ½ medium
Red Pepper 1 small
Yellow Pepper 1 small
Beef Tomato 1
Sweet Potato 1 small
Halloumi 250g
Olive Oil 2 tablespoons or 30ml
Wooden Skewers 4

PESTO INGREDIENTS

Fresh Basil 1 handful or 30g
Parmesan or Parmigiano
Reggiano Cheese 35g
Pine Nuts 1 small handful
or 30g
Olive Oil 4 Tablespoons
or 60ml
Lemon 1
Himalayan Rock Salt 1 pinch
Ground Black Pepper
1 generous pinch

PREPARE THE STACKS

Preheat the oven to 180°C / gas mark 4.

Remove the ends from the courgette, peel and cut lengthways into 4 slices. Cut the peppers into quarters and remove the seeds and core. Take a thin slice from each end of the beef tomato and discard. Slice the remaining tomato into 4 slices. Peel the sweet potato and slice lengthways into 4 slices. Cut the halloumi into 8 slices.

COOK

Drizzle ½ a tablespoon of olive oil onto a baking tray (making sure the tray is covered). Place the sweet potato onto the tray leaving as much room around each piece as possible, then drizzle ½ a tablespoon of olive oil over the slices. Place in the oven for 10 minutes.

ASSEMBLE THE STACKS

Meanwhile make the stacks. Take a skewer and add 1 piece of red pepper; 1 slice of halloumi; 1 slice of courgette; 1 piece of yellow pepper; 1 slice of halloumi and finish with 1 slice of tomato. Repeat until you have made 4 x stacks. Once cooked, remove the tray from the oven and turn the potatoes over. Next place the skewered stacks on top of each potato to form a stack with the red pepper on the top. Then drizzle each stack with the remaining olive. Return to the oven and cook for 25 minutes.

MAKE THE PESTO

Remove the basil leaves from the stalks and discard the stalks. Roughly chop the cheese and put all the ingredients in the large blending container that accompanies the hand blender (cut the lemon in half and squeeze the juice directly into the container). Blitz for about 30 seconds

SERVE

Place 2 stacks on each plate and drizzle over the pesto dressing.

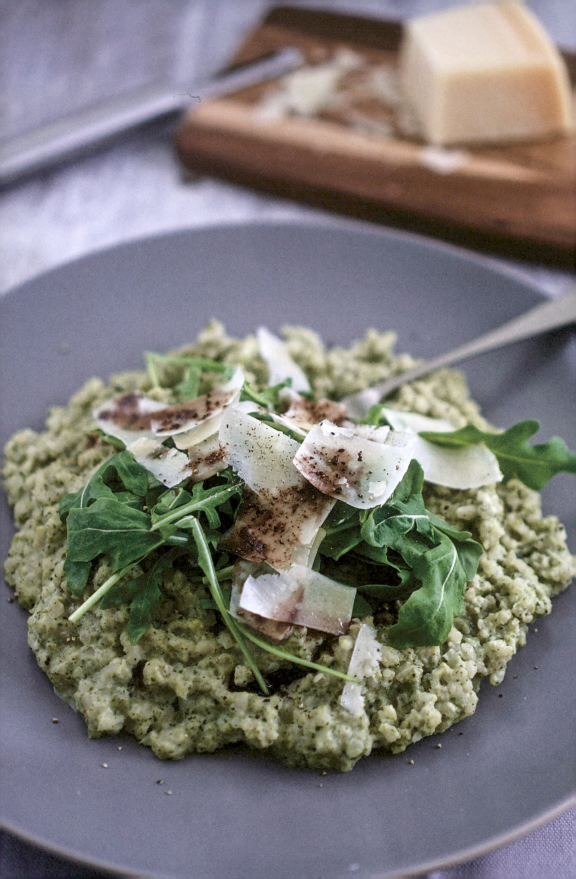

PURÉED PEA & MINT RISOTTO WITH WILD ROCKET & BALSAMIC

If I was ever trapped on a desert island and was only allowed one meal, this would be it. I don't like this recipe, I LOVE it, a disproportionate amount (you know the 'get a room' type love it). This is a 'must make' recipe as it's easy, nutritious and delicious. Chlorophyll rich rocket adds a peppery punch in flavour and nudges up the nutrition in the form of powerful phytonutrients, vitamins A, C, K, folate and calcium. Seriously, whoever said being healthy meant eating tasteless food needed to have tried this!

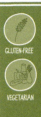

GLUTEN-FREE

VEGETARIAN

INGREDIENTS
Serves 2

Red onion ½ medium
Garlic 2 cloves
Parmesan or Parmigiano Reggiano Cheese 75g
Olive Oil 1 tablespoon or 15ml
Risotto Rice 200g
Boiling Water 600ml
Himalayan Rock Salt 2 pinches
Ground Black Pepper 2 generous pinch
Peas 100g (fresh or frozen)
Fresh Mint handful or 30g
Boiling Water 200ml (for the peas)
Crème Fraîche 50ml
Wild rocket large handful or 40g
Balsamic vinegar ½ tablespoon

PREPARE

Remove the ends and skin from the onion and garlic and dice into very small pieces. Using a vegetable peeler, slice the cheese into thin slivers.

COOK

Place the olive oil in a large pan and warm over a medium heat. Add the onion and garlic and cook for 5 minutes stirring frequently. Then add the rice and cook for a further 2 minutes, stirring constantly. Add 200ml of the boiling water, 1 pinch of salt and 1 pinch of pepper; reduce the heat and allow most of the water to absorb, stirring frequently. Keep adding 200ml of water at a time until all is absorbed and the rice is cooked (you may need to add a little more water, if the rice is not completely cooked at this stage). When cooked, add half the cheese, stir well and remove from the heat. Meanwhile place the peas in a small pan, cover with the boiling water (200ml) and boil for 5 minutes.

BLEND

Drain the cooked peas, place in the mixing container of a hand blender or the Super Blend or bullet style blender along with the mint and crème fraîche and blend for 30 seconds. Then add the pea and mint purée along with the remaining salt and pepper to the risotto and stir well.

SERVE

Pile the risotto onto a shallow bowl or plate, top with the rocket, cheese shavings and drizzle with balsamic vinegar.

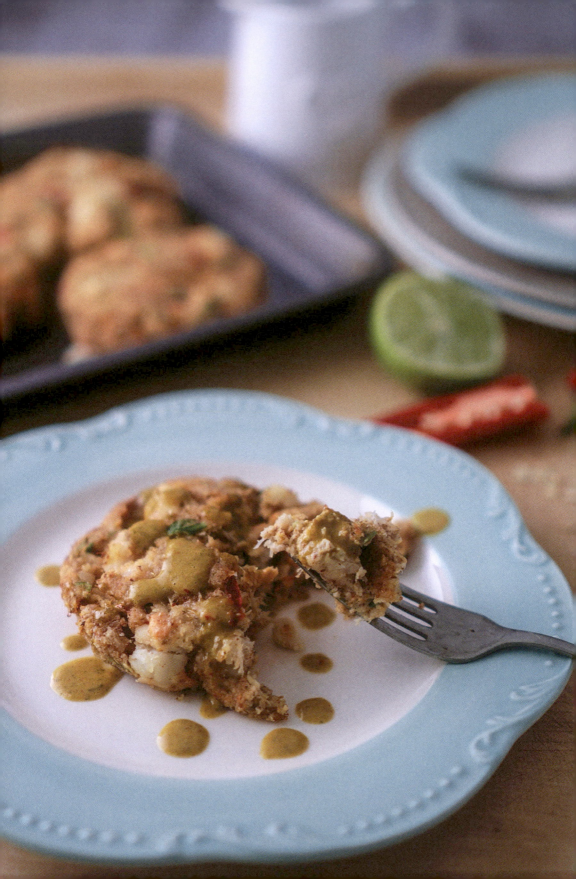

SWEET CHILLI FISHCAKES WITH A ZESTY LIME, CHILLI & CORIANDER DRESSING

If you've never made your own fresh fishcakes, I'm hoping this easy to make recipe will be your catalyst for change. Fish is so incredibly good for you that every health governing body in the world, suggests eating it at least 3 times a week. As well as heart-healthy mono and polyunsaturated fats, cod in particular is a significant source of omega-3 fatty acids and is without a doubt a true 'super food'. These tasty cakes are great served on their own, on a bed of fresh leaves or with some cheeky sweet potato wedges.

FISHCAKE INGREDIENTS

Serves 2

Sweet potato 1 medium
Garlic 2 cloves
Spring Onion 2 sprigs
Red Chilli 1 large
Cod Fillet 200g (without the skin)
Almonds 100g
Olive Oil 1 tablespoon or 15ml
Himalayan Rock Salt 1 pinch
Ground Black Pepper
1 generous pinch

DRESSING INGREDIENTS

Red Chilli 1 medium
Fresh Coriander small handful or 20g
Apple Cider Vinegar
1 tablespoon or 15 ml
Olive Oil 3 tablespoons or 45ml
Lime ½

PREPARE THE FISHCAKES

Preheat the oven to 180°C / gas mark 4.

Remove the ends from the sweet potato, peel and chop into chunks. Remove the ends and skin from the garlic. Remove the ends and outer layer from the spring onion and thinly slice. Remove the top and seeds from the red chilli and thinly slice. Cut the cod into small pieces. Using either the Super Blend; bullet style blender or a hand blender and container, blitz the almonds for 10-20 seconds until they turn into 'flour'. Place the sweet potato and garlic onto a baking tray, drizzle with the olive oil and mix, so all are coated, then place in the oven for 15 minutes stirring part way through.

COMBINE

Put the cooked sweet potato, garlic, almond 'flour', cod, spring onion, chilli, salt and pepper into a pan (set the baking tray to one side, but do not wash and do not turn the oven off) and gently mash using a potato masher, until everything is combined but the mixture still contains pieces of fish. Then using your (clean!) hands, divide the mixture into four, shape into 'burgers', then place on the baking tray and pop back in the oven. Cook for 20 minutes.

MIX THE DRESSING

Remove the top from the chilli, slice in half lengthways, remove the seeds and place in the mixing container of a hand blender (make sure the blade is already in). Add the other ingredients, squeezing the lime juice directly into the container. Blitz for 10-20 seconds.

SERVE

Gently remove the fishcakes from the tray and either enjoy on their own with the dressing, or serve them alongside a gorgeous salad.

GLUTEN-FREE

CONTAINS NUTS

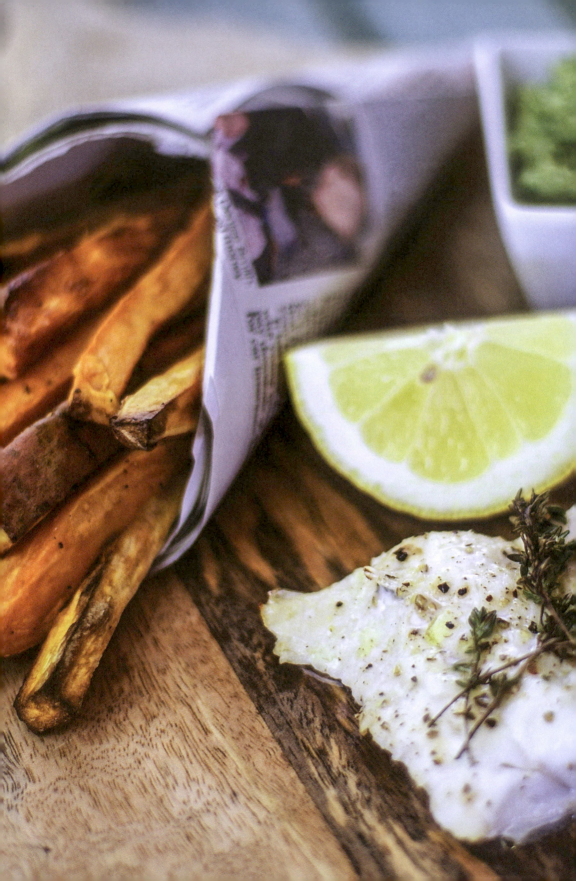

JASON'S CHEEKY FISH 'N' CHIPS WITH MINT PEA PURÉE

Fish 'n' Chips, the great British Friday night staple and a dish I'd find it hard to live without. The problem has always been the deep-frying of the fish, the batter and the way the chips are cooked. There is a way to have healthy Fish 'n' Chips and this is it! Plus it totally leaves the 'traditional' version begging when it comes to nutrition. The mint pea puree is so simple to make but will blow your mind with the first mouthful. Peas may be small in size but their nutrition is not to be underestimated, boasting valuable levels of vitamin A, C, B6 and a multitude of minerals including iron and magnesium. Come on people, it's time to give peas a chance!

GLUTEN-FREE

CONTAINS NUTS

INGREDIENTS

Serves 2

Sweet potato 2 large
Olive Oil 4 teaspoons or 60ml
Cod Fillet 2 approx150g–200g
Fresh Thyme 1 handful or 20g
Himalayan Rock Salt 2 pinches
Ground Black Pepper
2 generous pinches
Lemon 1

INGREDIENTS FOR THE MINT PUREE

Fresh or Frozen Peas 1 large handful or 80g
Fresh Mint Leaves 1 small handful or 20g

PREPARE THE CHIPS

Preheat the over to 200°C/gas mark 6.

Chop the ends off of the sweet potatoes and cut lengthways into 'chips' Drizzle half the olive oil into a baking tray, add a couple of pinches of salt and pepper and heat in the oven for 2 minutes. Add the sweet potatoes and toss to ensure they are coated in oil.

COOK

Place in the oven for 15 minutes.

PREPARE THE FISH

Drizzle the remaining olive oil over both pieces of fish (on both sides), season with a couple of pinches of pepper and place skin side down on a plate or board. Squeeze ½ of the lemon across both pieces and put the thyme on top.

COOK

When the potatoes have cooked for 15 minutes, add the fish to the baking tray skin side down and cook for a further 10 minutes.

BLEND THE PUREE

Meanwhile bring a pan of water to the boil and cook the peas for 3 –4 minutes. Then place the peas and mint leaves into the mixing container of a hand blender and squeeze in ¼ of the lemon juice. Blend until smooth (if you feel you need a little more moisture, add a drop of water).

SERVE

When the cod and sweet potatoes are cooked, place on a plate, add the pea puree, season the cod and chips with salt and pepper and add a final squeeze of lemon juice to the cod.

A ROUGH

WEEK IN

THE LIFE

OF THE 5:2

JUICE DIET

8

Please remember this is just a 'rough' guide of how a week *may* look, but there are so many variations that it would be virtually impossible to lay them all out in this book. Some of you may be veggie, others vegan, others who eat meat etc., so the meal suggestions may not float your boat and are simply suggestions. The one thing that will remain the same are the two days of juicing, how you live your other five days is up to you. Here is a 'rough' week in the life of a *5:2 Juice Diet System* and how I often live my week. Holidays will, of course, be different, along with special occasions that may come midweek, but essentially this is the outline for a system that will reap many rewards on the health and weight front, whilst at the same time, allowing you to be 'human' and join your friends and family for whatever takes your fancy! You may also choose to add some cheeky cappuccinos or lattes in there too, again it's your call.

MONDAY

ON WAKING: Herbal/Green Tea
or Hot Water and Lemon

9AM: Juice 1 — Power Plant

1PM: Juice 2 — Viva La Veggie

4PM: Juice 3 — Fennel Fury

7PM: Juice 4 — Pearfection

Monday and Tuesday are, as you'd expect, your 'juice fast' days. However, as I have mentioned many times, you can choose any two consecutive or non-consecutive days you wish. Personally, I switch from Monday & Tuesday to Tuesday & Wednesday at times. This decision is usually made by what I have left in the fridge from the weekend. I don't like food waste and so at times I eat on the Monday and juice on the Tuesday and Wednesday, but again this is your call. The recipes I have given here are from week one, but clearly you can slot in whatever juices from any other week.

TUESDAY

ON WAKING: Herbal/Green Tea
or Hot Water and Lemon

9AM: Juice 1 — Clean + Green

1PM: Juice 2 — Basil Blush

4PM: Juice 3 — Ginger Ninja

7PM: Juice 4 — Fresh + Wild

WEDNESDAY

ON WAKING: Herbal/Green Tea/Normal Tea/Coffee or Hot Water and Lemon

BREAKFAST: Juice or Smoothie

LUNCH: Super Salad or Smoothie

DINNER: Pea & Mint pureed Risotto with Wild Rocket & Balsamic

You will notice that I have included coffee in the equation. The reason for this is because this is essentially a *5:2 Juice Diet* and so what you do for the other five days is up to you. You may find that if you did a full 'juice fast' to launch you right into the *5:2 Juice Diet* way of life, you may well be off coffee anyway. However, if you are still a coffee head, feel free. There are many who will have a coffee on juice days too, this is not ideal, but if that's the only way you can see it through for those two days, then again, drink up.

You will also notice I have kept breakfast as a juice or smoothie. They say breakfast is the most important meal of the day and I agree. This is why I suggest that even on non 'juice fast' days you still keep the habit of a freshly extracted juice or smoothie for breakfast.

THURSDAY

ON WAKING: Herbal/Green Tea/Normal Tea/Coffee or Hot Water and Lemon

BREAKFAST: Juice or Smoothie

LUNCH: Super Salad

DINNER: Grilled Halloumi & Vegetable Stack, Drizzled with a Lemon Pesto Dressing

Once again we're keeping to 'clean' living and again kicking off the day with a nice juice or smoothie.

For lunch, either another juice/smoothie or a nice fresh salad (page 189 or 191). If the idea of a salad for lunch doesn't rock your world, then clearly you are free to have any Low H.I. (Human Intervention) meal (page 119 or 205).

Dinner tends to be a more substantial meal, so I have suggested something with a little more bite for the evening. Find a couple more examples here (page 197 or 203).

Again these are only suggestions and if you aren't following the *5:2 Juice Diet System*, but rather just the *5:2 Juice Diet* and don't care what you have for the other five days, then clearly have ANYTHING!

FRIDAY

ON WAKING: Herbal/Green Tea/Normal Tea/Coffee or Hot Water and Lemon

BREAKFAST: Juice or Smoothie

LUNCH: Super Salad

DINNER: Jasey's Fish 'n' Chips

Friday was always fish & chips night when I was growing up, so I have continued that tradition but with a much healthier version.

Once again we kick off the day with a freshly extracted juice/smoothie or, if you prefer, a nice omelette.

Lunch is something light but filling, so again a super food salad of some kind works well.

Dinner, as it's Friday, it's my version of Fish & Chips! This is an example and I am sure you won't want this every night. Once again, I'd rather biassedly like to recommend my *SUPER fast FOOD* book as it has over 100 Low H.I. 'Clean' recipes that will tantalize even the fussiest of taste buds. There are now many books containing beautiful, 'clean' food recipes and the internet is also a great place to seek out recipes too.

SATURDAY

ON WAKING: ANYTHING YOU LIKE

BREAKFAST: ANYTHING YOU LIKE

LUNCH: ANYTHING YOU LIKE

DINNER: ANYTHING YOU LIKE

This is what makes the *5:2 Juice Diet System* a programme anyone can follow. I have chosen the weekend as your 'human days' as these are the days we tend to need the most flexibility on the food front. I am aware that by calling them 'human days' I am implying that on the other days you aren't 'being human'. This can enforce the false belief that eating clean = no fun. This clearly isn't true as some of the tastiest food you'll ever eat is simple and clean, so please know I have only used the term 'human days' in relation to 'being human' and embracing all that life has to offer. This is why I have put ANYTHING YOU LIKE for Saturday & Sunday.

SUNDAY

ON WAKING: ANYTHING YOU LIKE

BREAKFAST: ANYTHING YOU LIKE

LUNCH: ANYTHING YOU LIKE

DINNER: ANYTHING YOU LIKE

With the danger of repeating myself again, please remember you are free to have anything you want on the other five non-fasting days. What I am hoping is that, after your five-day 'juice fast' to launch you into the *5:2 Juice Diet System*, you'll want to eat clean for at least three days a week.

THE
Q & A
SESSION

9

…If you don't find the answer you are looking for in this section, jump over to www.juicemaster.com or hit Facebook www.facebook.com/juicemasterltd as since the launch of this book, no doubt other questions have come up and been answered. Having said that, please make a point of reading this section as you will find most, if not all, of your 5:2 related questions here.

Q. YOU MENTIONED KICKING OFF WITH A FIVE DAY 'JUICE FAST' AND SAID TO READ 'HOW TO GO ABOUT' IN THE Q & A SESSION — SO HERE I AM?

A. There's a couple of ways you can do the 'launch' five days 'juice fast'.

1. Use the set **5lbs in 5 Days Juice Master Detox Diet** plan

2. Use the recipes in this book but **with a little adaptation**

Many of you reading this book will already have my *5lbs in 5 Days* book. If that's you, I would suggest re-reading the first 107 pages and cracking on with it. If you are either new to this or don't have said book, then clearly you'd have to get it. I am hesitant to say this, as it looks like I am trying to sell you another book when you have already invested in this one. However, the five-day *launch* 'juice fast' is just a suggestion and not part of the *5:2 Diet* as such, which is why it is a separate book and why, in order to do this *5:2 Juice Diet*, you don't have to buy it. You only need to get it should you choose to do the five-day *launch* and if you choose to do it using that particular plan. As mentioned, you don't have to do the five days using the specific *5lbs in 5 Days* book, you can simply use the recipes in this book with a slight adaptation. That slight adaptation is this: if you're going to use the recipes in this book, PLEASE HAVE *FIVE* JUICES A DAY. If you aren't going to use this book, and only want to have four a day, you can add some avocado or a banana to your morning and evening juices, as it is really important you get your fats in. If you own the *5lbs in 5 Days* app, I would really encourage you to watch the daily coaching videos, they will make all the difference. If perhaps you have never done a five-day 'juice fast' before, then even if you are using the adapted recipes in this book, I strongly advise you get the app if only for the coaching alone. You could then argue, I guess, that if you are getting the app for the coaching, you may as well use that plan! I cannot emphasise enough the momentum a full five days on juice will give you and I have no qualms in telling you to get the app in order to make sure you don't just *start* the 'launch', but you actually you complete it. Once again though, you don't have to get either that book or that app and can simply use the recipes in this book with the adaptations I have mentioned. If you don't get the book or app then PLEASE at the very least watch *Super Juice Me! The Big Juice Experiment* the night before you start, it will make doing the five days a lot easier, *www.superjuiceme.com*.

Q. DO YOU HAVE TO DO CONSECUTIVE DAYS OR CAN I DO ANY TWO DAYS A WEEK?

A. You are free to do any two days that work for you. Some choose to do two consecutive days, others non-consecutive days. In terms of weight loss and health benefits, there is no solid science to suggest it makes any difference. In terms of practicality, both work in their own ways and it will be up to you to decide which system fits your particular lifestyle. Some people choose to do two consecutive days and the ones who do, tend to pick Mondays and Tuesdays. This is because most find it easy to shop for their fruit and veg on a Sunday and find it's easier buying two days worth at once. Conversely, there are arguments for doing non-consecutive days too, the main one being you are only ever one day away from using your teeth! This was what led Dr Michael Mosley to choose non-consecutive days for his *5:2 Food Diet* concept, he always knew he could eat the following day and so it never really felt like a diet. I understand this psychology and it is why non-consecutive days work so well for many.

The choice is yours and as long as you do two full days of pure juice then you can safely say you are adhering to the principle. Each to their own is the conclusion here but personally I mix it up... because I'm out there!

Q. DO I HAVE TO STICK TO THE JUICES IN THE PLAN, OR CAN I SUPPLEMENT WITH OTHERS FROM YOUR OTHER PLANS AND BOOKS?

A. The juices in the plan have all been calculated for their calorie content. Clearly, depending on the size of the produce you buy, those calorie counts may change slightly. All of the science appears to point to 500 calories a day for women and 600 calories a day for men for optimum Intermittent Fasting results. Each of the juices in this plan are around 125/150 calories and so guarantee to meet this scientific criteria. This is why, for the purposes of the *5:2 Juice Diet*, it's best to stick to the suggested juices in this plan. Having said that, you are of course free to substitute other juices from my other books and plans, but make sure you don't make any of the 'smoothies' with yoghurt, bananas or avocados as they'll immediately put you top heavy on the calorie count. I have never been a fan of calorie counting in any way and it seems extremely alien to be doing it now. The only reason for this is because there is a great deal of research now using these numbers. As a rough guide, a 420ml vegetable based juice comes in at around 150 calories and an avocado smoothie of the same size around 250 calories. You really don't need to get too bogged down with these exact numbers and two days of freshly extracted juice per week will do your waistline and health wonders, even if you go slightly over on the calorie front. I would also add that humans come in all sorts of shapes and sizes and the amount of movement each person does varies massively. If you are 6ft 4in and play rugby all day, then adding shed loads of avocados and bananas to your juices would be deemed an intelligent thing to do. It is extremely difficult when writing a book of this nature to cover all bases as there will always be a need to use your common sense and be flexible. The vast majority can do the *5:2 Juice Challenge* as it's laid out in this book and won't need to adjust, however there will be some people who do, so please use your common sense and listen to your body!

Q. WILL THEY STILL BE OF GOOD NUTRITIONAL VALUE IF I MAKE THEM IN ADVANCE AND DRINK THROUGHOUT THE DAY?

A. Freshly made and drunk within one hour of making will always be the best. Having said that, very rarely does this model fit into the average person's hectic life. Not only that, but most people really don't want to wash their juicer four times a day. With this in mind there are a couple of options to make life easier:

1.   Make all the juices for the day, put them into

flasks, dark bottles or 'boosters'. Keep them as cold as possible and don't allow oxygen or light in. These will keep nicely for the day.

2. Make all the juices the night before the two-day 'fast', put the first two in flasks and pop into the fridge for the morning of day one and simply freeze the rest. You can then remove the afternoon juices for day one in the morning, pop them in the fridge and, by the afternoon, they should be ready to drink. That night remove the frozen juices for day two, place in the fridge and they'll be ready the next day. Unlike cooking, freezing preserves the nutrients so hardly anything is lost. Make all your juices in a slow 'cold press' juicer. The slower the juicer the less heat friction applied and the longer your juice will keep. These types of juicers are becoming more and more popular as people become much more aware of the different types of juicers and what they can offer. For the best results, other than making 100 per cent fresh and drinking right away, would be to make in a 'cold press' juicer and then freeze. I am, however, aware that the vast majority of people have 'fast' juicers (and often for good 'I just need to juice and go' reasons) and juicing in this type of juicer

and freezing is still extremely good! If you do own a 'cold press' juicer, Sunday's are a great day for making a batch. Because freezing doesn't destroy the nutrients, you can even make a whole month's worth, if you have the freezer space. For a list of what juicers are best see (PAGE 239/CHAPTER 10).

Q. CAN I MAKE ALL THE JUICES IN A 'NUTRIBULLET', 'NUTRININJA', 'RETRO SUPER BLEND' OR SIMILAR?

A. No! Contrary to what the advertising says, the Nutribullet is NOT a juicer – it's a blender. So too is the Nutrininja and any other 'bullet looking' BLENDER. I have used all of the above and all are great blenders, but none of them are juicers. They are in essence like a mini 'Vitamix', but they're not juicers. In order to do the *5:2 Juice Diet* you need a *juicer*... not a blender. If you wish to add things like avocados/ bananas and so on then getting one of these blender bad boys is a great investment, I just wanted to clear up any confusion about the difference between the two machines. A juicer extracts the *juice* contained with the fibres of the fruit or vegetable and a blender *blends* it all together. The point of juicing is to extract the juice as it's the part of the fruit and vegetable which feeds the body, fibre cannot penetrate through the intestinal wall, so contrary to popular 'juice skeptic' belief, you won't be losing anything on the nutrition front. In fact, because the juicer has extracted the life by giving juice from the fibres, it is more bio-available – meaning more of the nutrients get to where they are needed.

Q. SO EXACTLY WHAT IS THE BEST JUICER TO GET?

A. Not an easy question to answer as there are now so many different models on the market today, all promising different things. All you need to know is that there are 3 types of juicer – slow, fast and low-induction. All have their merits, but the juice made in slow juicers, in my opinion, is of much better nutritional quality. This type of juicing creates less heat friction and more soluble fibre is retained, which makes for a more filling juice. The pulp is always usually bone dry, so saves you money on produce. The downside is they are called slow juicers for a reason! Having said that there is, at the time of writing this, a new kid on the slow juicing block – the Retro Cold Press juicer. *www.retrojuicer.com* this not only looks great (they have a Brit and Pink edition to die for!), but it makes an incredible juice and you can fit whole apples in. The most popular juicers are fast juicers and there's no prize for guessing why – they're fast! There are some great models on the market right now but it's ever changing so I won't pinpoint any particular one here. Simply go to *www.juicemaster.com* for my latest recommendations. I have dedicated a mini chapter on 'So What Juicer Is Best, Jase?' (PAGE 239/CHAPTER 10) and advise you to take a look at it so you can get the right juicer... *for you.*

Q. WHAT'S THE BEST WAY TO GET MENTALLY PREPARED?

A. Watch the film *Super Juice Me! The Big Juice Experiment*. It documents eight people who went on a journey of drinking nothing but juice for 28 days. Trust me, after you watch this two days will seems like a piece of cake (so to speak). Go to *www.superjuiceme.com*.

Q. I HAVE DONE ONE OF YOUR FULL JUICE DIETS, IS IT OK TO JUMP ON THIS DIRECTLY AFTERWARDS?

A. YES! And YES again. The whole idea for many when they jump on any of my 'juice diets' is not simply to get into that little black dress or smaller waist jeans, but to kick start a healthy lifestyle and to keep whatever weight they have lost off permanently. There are, of course, many ways to make sure you don't gain the weight back, but the *5:2 Juice Diet* is one of the most effective. It also means you don't really have to think, simply juice for two days a week and eat whatever you like for the other five. Hopefully after you've finished one of my juice diets you won't want junk food on the other five days but instead good wholesome food. But even if you don't, juicing for two days a week goes a long way to balance any indiscretions!

Q. CAN I DRINK ANY TEA OR COFFEE DURING JUICING DAYS?

A. There is no reason why you can't have one or two cups of tea of coffee per day on juicing days. It's not ideal and for ideal results you should drink only herbal teas or hot water and lemon. Having said this, if you are a coffee drinker and you really don't want to stop, then the last thing you want is a headache two days a week! So feel free to indulge. However, what I will say is, make sure they are your standard Americano coffees and not calorie packed latte's or cappuccinos.

Q. CAN I EAT ANYTHING ELSE ON THE JUICING DAYS?

A. As I mentioned in the book, you can eat some fruit *if* you can't juice for whatever reason, but essentially no you shouldn't have anything other than your juices on 'juice fast' days.

Q. WHAT CAN I EAT ON THE OTHER FIVE DAYS?

A. Anything you like. Ideally you would have a juice for breakfast for at least three of the other days and eat good whole foods, but this is the real world and many will want to eat all sorts of things. This is why the *5:2 Juice Diet* works for so many as it gives them total flexibility for five days a week, whilst providing them with the tools for steady, permanent weight loss. I have included some recipes from my *SUPER fast FOOD* cookbook in this book and ideally for at least three of the other five days you'd eat 'clean', as it were. This will go a long way to making sure you maintain good health and any weight loss achieved before you started this or whilst you've been doing it. If you ever get that particular book not only does it have over 100 of the finest 'clean' recipes, but it also has my *Super Charge Me! 7-Day Food Plan*, which maps out a 'day in the life of'.

Q. CAN I DRINK ALCOHOL ON 'FAST' DAYS?

A. Nope.

Q. I'M GOING ON HOLIDAY, HOW DO I DO CONTINUE TO DO THE 5:2 Juice Diet?

A. Many will choose their holiday as a holiday from the *5:2 Juice Diet* too. I mentioned at the start of this book the importance of CC (Consistent Commitment) and that what you do *most* of the time determines your weight and health. If you holiday for even up to six weeks a year (yes, that would be nice!) and you live by the *5:2 Juice Diet* for the rest of the year, you are still in CC mode. Six weeks out of 52 and you're still in the 'most of the time' ratio. If you also join in with my four global guided juice 'fasts', then you've gone way over your juice quota, even if you don't juice at all on your holiday weeks. Having said all of that, many people don't want to break the routine and wish to keep on 5:2 whilst on their hols. You can take your juicer, but that's a little extreme and not really necessary. Allow fruit to be your 'juice' while you are away, as effectively most of it is. Watermelon is 99 per cent nutritional water and even an avocado is over 80 per cent, as too is a banana. The humble banana is only around 100 calories and a good size avocado is about 200/250. So if you do wish to keep the 5:2 going whilst away, let fruit be thy solution and leave your juicer at home.

Q. CAN I EXERCISE ON THE 'JUICE FAST' DAYS?

A. YES! There is no reason why you need to stop exercising when having only fresh juice for that day. When I first did my seven-day juice cleanse (to test it before writing the *7lbs in 7 Days* book), I found I had *more* energy to exercise. On day six I even ran a half marathon and felt I could have gone on way longer. At my juice-only retreats we have four juices a day and provide around five hours worth of exercise, ranging from morning hill walks, to rebounding, fitness classes and yoga. We don't even have our first juice until 10. 30am as we encourage people to be 'fat burning', as opposed to 'sugar burning'. It's also one of the reasons people have such incredible weight loss success on the retreats. Clearly, everyone is different and I will just point out that if this is brand new to you and you are moving away from a diet of refined fat, salt, sugar and caffeine, you may well feel incredibly tired on your first couple of 'juice fast' days. This is often caused by 'withdrawal', which often gets confused with 'detoxing'. The message is an obvious one, but I have to add it just in case, LISTEN TO YOUR OWN BODY. *You* will know if you have the energy to exercise, *you* will know if you are feeling faint, *you* are the best person to judge whether you should exercise or not. What I will say though is that, through my 15 years of experience in this field, I personally have no issue with exercising on juice-only days, any more than I have on non-juice days. Sometimes you're in the mood and other times you're not, often irrespective of what you are eating, or not, that day. We tend to over analyse everything the second we do anything out of the norm, like juice for a day, and immediately everything we feel is because of the fact we are on juice. Other days when we are eating 'normally' we may feel an energy slump but just put it down to the day, if we're on juice it's always down to that fact. You'll have energy days and non-energy days, whether you are consuming juice or food, that's just the human body. I say, if you can at all, embrace exercise on 'juice fast' days, but always consult your doctor first (I am obligated to write that and yes it bugs me that I have to, I mean you're not a numpty are you?!)

Q. ARE THERE ANY NEGATIVE SIDE EFFECTS TO WATCH OUT FOR?

A. NO, not usually. However, you should always listen to your body (not your mind as that can play many tricks!) If you feel extremely faint, or that 'something is just not quite right' then use your intuition and stop. Then see your doctor as there is no reason for this to make you ill, unless you are genuinely allergic to a certain fruit or vegetable. As with anything, listen to how you feel and act accordingly.

Q. CAN I DO THE 5:2 JUICE DIET IF PREGNANT OR IF TRYING TO CONCEIVE?

A. As with all these things, you need to consult your doctor. We live in a world where we have to consult our doctors if we want to consume freshly extracted vegetable juices for a couple of days in the week, but if you fancy stuffing pizza, crisps, chocolate, muffins, sweets, ice-cream, cola etc. etc. you don't need to consult anyone!

Q. CAN I BUY SHOP BOUGHT JUICES TO DO THE 5:2 JUICE DIET ?

A. NO! The reason I am so adamant about this is because the pasteurized/cooked juice you buy in a bottle or carton in the shops is not the same as freshly extracted juice. You also don't know how many calories you'd be consuming, a seemingly very important aspect of IF and CR. There are now plenty of 'cold pressed' juices in bottles, but even these are not the same as the real, freshly extracted variety. You also don't know the quality of the produce used. As you are living on nothing but juice for two days a week, the quality of the produce is extremely important. This is why I will almost always juice fresh on the two days, or juice in advance and freeze the juices for the days I need them. On occasion yes I will have a 'cold pressed' juice from a shop in a bottle, but this is only to get me out of trouble if, for whatever reason, I don't have access to fresh.

Q. CAN I DRINK ALCOHOL ON 'JUICE FAST' DAYS?

A. NOPE!

Q. WON'T MY BODY JUST GO INTO 'STARVATION MODE' AND SO HANG ONTO FAT AND MAKE ME FATTER IN THE LONG RUN?

A. The simple answer is NO, not at all. Because the 'fasting' is a) short lived each week and b) not really actual 'fasting' in the true starvation sense of the word, your body will burn energy from fat stores but won't eat muscle tissue. There has been research done that shows that Intermittent Fasting does not suppress metabolism. So please do not be concerned that it will cause more of a 'fat memory' in the long run, because it won't.

Q. I'M ALREADY THIN BUT WANT THE OTHER HEALTH BENEFITS OF THE 5:2 JUICE DIET , IS IT OK FOR ME TO DO?

A. Only you can really advise yourself on this one. Being too thin is often more harmful than being too fat and the last thing I would want is for you to become a 'juicarian' and get too thin. If you are already slim/thin I would say a 6:1 rather than *5:2 Juice Diet* is about as much as you should do, but swapping your breakfast for a juice each day, will reap many benefits. You could also blend some avocado and banana in a couple of juices as a way of increasing the calorie content. There is certainly no harm at all going pure 'live' juice/smoothie for two days a week, but if you are thin already then increase to around 1,200 calories a day.

Q. CAN I DO MORE THAN TWO DAYS OF JUICE-ONLY EACH WEEK?

A. YES! If you want to do a 4:3 rather than a 5:2, feel free. I have one extremely famous client who does three days of juicing every single week and she is in the best shape of her life. You cannot, nor should, live on juice alone, and as an ongoing thing, the maximum you should do is three days juice four days food. Yes you can do one-off longer juice cleanses, but as on ongoing weekly way of life, please keep to these guidelines. If you are severely overweight and want to do the full *Super Juice Me! 28-Day Juice Plan* before going to 5:2, please see your doctor first.

Q. I HEAR YOU DELIVER THE 5:2 DIRECT TO YOUR DOOR, BUT IT SEEMS EXPENSIVE?

A. If you are ever hit with the lazy brush and fancy a

helping hand with making your juices, then you can choose the very easy way and get all of your 5:2 juices delivered to your door. However, though this isn't the cheapest option, it completely takes the hassle out of doing it at home. No need to shop, juice, or clean, we'll do everything for you. We use only the best produce and then we cold press and blast freeze to lock in the nutrients. We then put them into darkened bottles to prevent any light or oxygen getting to the juice. You take delivery whenever you like, and simply pop them in your freezer until you're ready to use. Like I said, it's not the cheapest option in the world, but I have learnt in life you get what you pay for. There are many juice delivery companies now, but not all are built the same and I like to call ours 'reassuringly priced'. The cheapest option, of course, is making them yourself at home, but in today's busy world, every now and then it's nice to have someone else make them for you! *www.juicemasterdelivered.com.*

SO WHAT JUICER IS BEST, JASE?

NOT THE EASIEST QUESTION TO ANSWER ANYMORE, BUT HERE GOES...

10

THE
JUICER
REVOLUTION

If there was a list of the top ten questions I get asked most frequently, then 'What juicer should I get?' is probably at first, with 'But what about the fibre?' and 'Isn't it all just sugar?' coming in strongly at numbers two and three. The answer to the number one question used to be easy, but times have changed and the juicer market is as swamped and confusing as most other markets.

When I first set out on my mission to 'Juice The World', over 15 years ago now, the range of juice extractors was hardly long – in fact it is safe to say it was pretty non-existent. If, and it was a very big *if*, you could find a juicer for sale in a regular electrical store (internet shopping hadn't really started at this time, and even if you did find anything you wanted to buy on the www, people just didn't trust putting giving their credit card details – my how things have changed), all you would have found was an extremely cheap, flimsy, small juicer. It would have had a tiny kidney shaped feeder for your fruits and vegetables and an extremely small pulp container. You would have had to chop all your fruit and veg into extremely small pieces and spent an age making a juice. If you wanted to make juice for a few of you, forget it, the machine would often block after making a single juice. You then would have had all the fun of the fair cleaning the thing, which was no easy task. Back then of course, the people who manufactured juicers hadn't thought about how long it may take someone to clean it, actually they hadn't really thought about the juicing process as a whole! This was probably due to the market being so tiny, not even one per cent of the UK, for example, owned a juicer at that time. My mission was, and still is today, to make a juicer and blender as common as a kettle and toaster in every kitchen globally. This goal is now not that far off as juicers and blenders are now commonplace and I like to think I may have had a little something to do with this. However, the point I am making is that back then I used to tell people to just 'get a juicer', now of course it's all about 'yes, but which one?'

Luckily juicing has moved on from the nightmare of juicers past and 21st century juicing is here to stay. Like most things in our fast paced 21st century world, speed is key for a lot of people. Juice extractors have essentially gone 'broadband' and the vast majority now come with a wide chute, which usually allows for two or three apples to be juiced whole – no chopping, no peeling, no hassle! This is something I dreamt of when I first started juicing. However, not all wide-funnel juicers are built the same. There are many coming in, 'off the shelf' from places like Asia, and big companies are simply adding their name to, often inferior, juicers. Many are very poorly made and lack the ability to actually juice. Yes you can *get* juice from them, but often the pulp contains as much juice as the juice itself. When you buy a juice extractor you need a machine that does 'exactly what it says on the tin' (so to speak), i.e. *extract* the *juice* efficiently from the fibres.

AND THE BEST JUICER
IN THE WORLD IS...

This is not the easiest question to answer because the best juicer in the world hasn't even been invented yet. As I have mentioned, I have been juicing for over 15 years and I have seen some great strides in juicing machines, but I have yet to find that all illusive 'Self-Cleaning Juicer'! This is the holy grail of juicers and although we may be quite a way from an automatic self-cleaning juicer, I have good intelligence informing me that the 'semi-self-cleaning juicer' is just around the corner. By the time you read this book the 'one click, semi-self-cleaning' technology may be here and if so, I would say this is probably the juicer you want to get, especially if this is your first outing to the juicing world. If it's not out yet, or the rumours were just that, rumours, then the best juicer to get is simple. In my first ever book I set out what the best exercise in the world is, the answer is simply – *the one you will do.* The same is now true of juicers. The best juicer in world is quite simply the one *you* will use, the one that suits *your* needs and, because looks do matter, the one that you feel will look coolest in your kitchen!

Currently there are three types of juicer to choose from:

- **Fast (Centrifugal)**

- **Slow (Cold Press or Masticating)**

- **Low-Induction**

FAST JUICERS

These are by far the most common types of juicer on the market. Fast, or 'centrifugal' juicers, as they are otherwise known, make up the vast majority of juicers sold in the world today. Most have very wide chutes, meaning you can put whole apples in and are extremely fast at juicing. There isn't a great deal to choose from these days in terms of performance, but you do tend to get what you pay for, I call it 'reassuringly priced'. If you see a wide funnel juicer at £40, there's usually a good reason it's just £40. We tend to spend a great deal of money on nights out, pay per view TV, alcohol, junk food and so on, but the second you ask someone to invest decent money in a juicer – something which can potentially help them live a long and disease-free existence – and cries of 'That's too expensive' soon follow. I used to buy two to three packets of cigarettes a day, on today's prices, that's over £20… *a day!* If I had smoked for 40 years of my life it would amount to over £300,000. The average person in the UK spends over £140,000 in their lifetime on alcohol, and £2,620 a year on takeaways. People aged between 25 to 34 are the biggest consumers of fast food, spending over £200 a month on the stuff (over 24 takeaways a month). Once you start to look at the numbers, which don't even take into account the money spent on medication to treat many of the health conditions these things often spawn, the investment in a juicer and blender starts to look very attractive indeed! Fast juicers, are not only the most common, but the best value too. This is why, especially if this is your first introduction to juicing, I would say this is the type of juicer you want to get. They are the easiest to use, quickest, easiest to clean and now, they even look cool too. Even the top players in this field, at time of writing this – Philips, Sage and Retro – will all set you back less than £200. The Retro Super Fast Juicer is the newest of all these and not only do they look as cool as hell – they are what they say – super fast to use and also to clean! I would also say, at this time, the Retro Super Fast juicer is the best value for what you get in this sector (*www.retrojuicer.com*). However, like mobile phones or any other technology, the juice extractor market is ever changing and new innovations are coming in thick and fast, so check out *www.juicemaster.com* for my up to date recommendations.

SLOW JUICERS

Slow juicers are also known as 'masticating' or 'cold press' juicers and tend to be more expensive and, as the name suggests, slower to use. However, when it comes to price again, you tend to get what you pay for. Even though they cost more, the quality of the juice is quite literally out of this world. Slow juicers extract the juice at *much* slower speeds and therefore don't create the heat friction that many fast juicers do. The pulp left behind is also often bone dry, meaning that if you are going to juice a lot, you'll save money on produce as more of the juice is extracted and not left in the pulp container. Having said that, there are now slow juicers that have whole chutes, meaning you can put whole apples in, making the process of 'cold press' juicing slightly faster. I say 'slightly' because even with a whole chute for apples, many still only move at 65–150 rpms, so will always be much slower than the 15,000 rpm fast juicers. The advantages of a 'cold press' juicer are three fold:

1. **Better quality juice**

2. **Better motor that lasts**

3. **Dry pulp so you save money on produce**

The main movers in this field are juicers like the Green Star and Matstone to name just a couple. The Green Star produces an extremely smooth and nutritious juice, but is really expensive and, like many slow juicers, a complete nightmare to clean. However, there are new 'upright' slow juicers like the Hurom and Oscar 930 and these are slightly cheaper and produce a wonderful juice. At the time of writing, the Retro Cold Press upright juicer is the new, slick, juicing kid on the block and seems to be stealing all the headlines. Not only because they produce a great juice, leave dry pulp and you can put a whole apple in, but they are simply the coolest juicers on the market (go to *www.retrojuicers.com* and you'll see what I mean). However, the slow juicer market is ever-changing so, see what's hot in the 'cold press' juicer market right now, jump to *www.juicemaster.com*.

LOW-INDUCTION JUICERS

These are the 'half way house' between slow and fast juicers. The 'Godfather of Fitness' and 'juicing guru' Jack LaLanne was one of the first to bring out a juicer of this nature. It was named after him and the 'Jack LaLanne Power Juicer' went on to become the best selling juicer in the US for over a decade. Sadly Jack passed away at the age of 96 and I was asked to try and fill his incredible boots. They changed the juicer slightly, but it was still a 'low-induction' juicer and they renamed it Jason Vale's Fusion Juicer. This type of juicer juices at speeds of about 3,000 rpm, so much slower than a 'fast' juicer but not as slow as a 'cold press' or 'slow' juicer – it's the middle ground, so to speak. However, what I soon discovered was that if someone was used to using a fast juicer and then switched to a Fusion, they were often left disappointed. As my name was written all over the juicer, it was me who personally got the abuse from those who thought the juicer was a pile of crap and not working properly. The only reason they thought this was because they were comparing it to their previous fast juicer, a completely different kind of machine. It would be like comparing a Fiat 500 and a Mini Cooper S, both get you from A to B but with different engines and both having their own unique upside. It's whether or not that upside is also *your* upside. If you like being economical, then the Fiat is for you, if you want speed, then it's the Mini Cooper. The truth is, the Fusion juicers low-induction motor is slower to use and takes a little getting used to, but it does indeed produce a superior juice. It was also much cheaper, in many cases, than the fast juicer. I thought this ticked all the boxes and was happy to put my name to it – you got better quality juice than a fast juicer, it was quicker to use than a slow juicer and it was relatively cheap. What I didn't account for was the fact that, because it looked like a fast juicer, people wanted it to perform exactly like a fast juicer and, when comparing the two machines, it seems speed was what they wanted over anything else. Contrary to what people make up in their head, I never owned the Fusion juicer and, like Philips before it, I simply put my name to it and got very, very little in return (again contrary to popular made-up belief). The reason I did put my name to it was that I was incredibly honoured to be asked by the big Americans to take over from the incredible Jack laLanne and I honestly thought the juicer was the best of all worlds. I still think the Fusion juicer fills that gap, but it appears it's a gap most don't want or understand. I have removed my name from this juicer and, from what I know, it's now been discontinued. You can still buy them here and there and I still stand by the fact that, for the money, they produce one hell of an amazing quality juice. I guess it's like the Betamax and VHS (yes I am showing my age here) battle for the video tape years ago. Despite the Sony Betamax tape being far superior to VHS, better quality and smaller than the VHS tape or recorder, the chunky VHS won and Betamax went into rapid decline never to be heard of again. We may see low-induction juicing again, but perhaps with such wonderful fast and 'cold press' juicers, people want either one or the other – not the in-betweener, that seemed, on the surface, to be the answer. Like the Betamax before it, perhaps the Fusion juicer may be assigned to the history books.

This is why I now say the best juicer to get is, 'the one you will use'! So pick a juicer that's right for *you* and *your* needs, not necessarily what's new on that market. Having said that, if this 'one click semi-self-cleaning' juicer becomes a reality, I'll be 'clicking to basket' quicker than you can say juice me up baby!

BUT WHAT JUICER DO YOU USE, JASON?

Over the years I have personally used many, many different juicers but the one I have come back to time and time again, is the Philips 1861. Unfortunately, despite me wanting to buy the rights from Philips for this machine, Philips decided to discontinue it. They then reinvented the juicer with an upside down bowl so you could see the juice being made and pulp hidden. Great idea on the surface, but if you are juicing for a few people, the juicer gets clogged as there's no separate pulp container. I will never, ever understand why Philips stopped making the

1861 as every juicer they have brought out since, in my opinion, just isn't as good. Now, before you jump on ebay looking for one of these, the good news is something has come along to take its place and I now use this one a lot of the time – the Retro Super Fast Juicer. I also use the Retro Cold Press when I have more time. I am a firm believer that if you are only going to have one juice a day – do it right. That means organic where possible and made in a slow juicer. This isn't always convenient and at times, speed is everything, which is why I use different machines depending on the time I have available, I also use the Fusion here and there to mix it up! I will point out that the reason I am such a fan of Retro at the moment is they are, as I have mentioned, the coolest juicing kids on the block *and* they are great juicers. I'm an aesthetic person and they just look great in the kitchen. My mission is for people to *use* their juicer, not just buy one, and you're much more likely to leave it out on the work surface, primed and ready for use, if it looks good – and boy these look GOOD! I also have a Retro Super Blend, it's like a Nutribullet type blender, only again it looks SO GOOD, as well as the fact it matches my 'cold press' and fast juicer. These are the juicers *I* use, but may well not be the juicers for *your* needs. Do the research and find what *you* like and what fits with *your* kitchen.

JOIN THE JUICE

REVOLUTION

11

There is a 'Juice Revolution' happening and I'm guessing now you've read this book, you're about to be part of it. For the past 15 years I have been on a mission to 'Juice The World' and I have seen this 'Juice Revolution' unfold before my very eyes. *Fresh* juicing is no longer seen as a fad and millions of people all over the world do some kind of 'juice fast' on a regular basis – I am one of them. As I mentioned at the start of the book, I do four 'juice fasts' a year, varying in length from five days to 14. People put their car in for a service and it always baffles me that don't do the same with their body – the most important vehicle they'll ever own. So as well as committing to the *5:2 Juice Diet*, why not commit to joining in with '*Jason Vale's Big Juice Challenge*' every season. It's all free and thousands of people join in. Funnily enough as I write this page over 20,000 people from 124 countries are taking part in one right now, as too am I. I am actually at my retreat in Portugal and shooting daily videos to bring everyone together and encourage people all the way. If you want to know more, then join my juicy community, you can do so in many ways:

FACEBOOK:

www.facebook.com/juicemasterltd

www.facebook.com/superjuiceme

TWITTER:

@juicemaster

JUICE TUBE!

www.youtube.com/user/juicemasterjasonvale

INSTAGRAM

@jasonvale

MAIN WEBSITES:

www.juicemaster.com

www.superjuiceme.com

www.juicemasterdelivered.com

www.juicyoasis.com

www.juicymountain.com